Environment, Economy, and Health in African Marginal Communities

Environment, Economy, and Health in African Marginal Communities

Edited by Aderemi Suleiman Ajala

LEXINGTON BOOKS
Lanham • Boulder • New York • London

Published by Lexington Books
An imprint of The Rowman & Littlefield Publishing Group, Inc.
4501 Forbes Boulevard, Suite 200, Lanham, Maryland 20706
www.rowman.com

86-90 Paul Street, London EC2A 4NE

British Library Cataloguing in Publication Information Available

Library of Congress Cataloging-in-Publication Data

Library of Congress Cataloging-in-Publication Data
Names: Ajala, Aderemi Suleiman, editor.
Title: Environment, economy, and health in African marginal communities / edited by Aderemi Suleiman Ajala.
Description: Lanham : Lexington Books, 2023. | Includes bibliographical references and index.
Identifiers: LCCN 2023019200 (print) | LCCN 2023019201 (ebook) | ISBN 9781666939866 (cloth) | ISBN 9781666939873 (epub)
Subjects: LCSH: Health services accessibility--Environmental aspects--Africa--Congresses. | Health services accessibility--Economic aspects--Africa--Congresses. | Marginality, Social--Health aspects--Africa--Congresses. | Poor--Medical care--Africa--Congresses. | Public health--Africa--Congresses.
Classification: LCC RA418.3.A35 E57 2023 (print) | LCC RA418.3.A35 (ebook) | DDC 362.1086/94096--dc23/eng/20230623
LC record available at https://lccn.loc.gov/2023019200
LC ebook record available at https://lccn.loc.gov/2023019201

Contents

List of Tables and Figure

TABLES

FIGURE

Acknowledgments

The most interesting aspect of editorial is the wide-ranging contributions from different authors from diverse backgrounds. Through this, the editor has a wider view of the research concerns covered in the editorial. Being a product of such relationship, this edited book enjoyed deep and productive engagements from all the contributors. I am therefore incredibly thankful to all the contributors.

Alexander von Humboldt Foundation, Germany, provided a grant to organize a colloquium in Nigeria in June 2022. Papers presented at the colloquium were selected for this publication. The foundation also supported the review and editing of the selected papers. Lexington Press also supported this with a publication grant. And the Department of Archaeology and Anthropology, University of Ibadan, Nigeria, provided an initial intellectual and institutional home for the conception and delivery of the ideas in this book. The combined effects of these two institutions no doubt made it possible to get this edited book published.

I also must mention the editorial board and anonymous reviewers for Lexington Books. I remain ever grateful for believing in this work and repackaging my ideas. I enjoyed the meticulous and painstaking processes involved in the publication of the book.

Chapter 1

Issues on Environment, Economy, and Health in African Marginal Communities

Aderemi Suleiman Ajala

Human health-care systems are mostly influenced by the twin factors of environment and economy. Specifically, the conceptualization of health care, the nature and type of health care, and access to health care in terms of location, availability, and affordability are dependent on the environment and economy. While the naturality of the environment is in itself a health-care challenge for human beings, the interaction, involving human negotiation within the environment in a bid to create culture, is another critical challenge for human health. Thus, human interactions on environment involve the human recognition of available resources, both material and non-materials, the possibility of harnessing the identified resources, appropriating values and importance of those resources, refining the resources to desirable usefulness, and the eventual utilization of the resources as consumable products. Within these interactions, human beings negotiate a shift and balance with the environment in materialists' perspective mostly in form of economic activities. Thus, human interaction with the environment defines health risks, readiness to take health clues, utilization patterns of health-care systems, and belief in functionality of the available health-care systems. These health concerns are determined by the nature of the environment, whether posing sufficient threats or not; the knowledge of the population, whether capable of recognizing and developing the resources available for maintaining healthy living in the environment or not; and the capacity of the population to reprocess the environment so as to make it healthy through the process of technology. The extent to which these forces are deployed categorizes societies or/and communities into health-care accessibility. While substantial research evidences are available on the interplay of those variables in accessible and non-marginal communities, in-accessible and marginal communities, like pastoral bands, fishing communities, quarry and mining sites, itinerant commuters, refugee camps, war-devastated communities, manufacturing sites, naturally alienated communities, and remote farm settlements, are yet to be widely covered in health research. Thus, this international colloquium focuses on cultural interaction among environment, economy, and health in marginal communities. A *marginal community* is defined as a community of human groups that is difficult to access for health-care intervention. Difficulty in access is defined by remoteness of the community, stressful economic production, small-scale population, and poor infrastructural facilities, among others.

In recognition of the above, the Alma Ata Declaration enunciated the Universal Access to Healthcare System since 1978 (WHO, 1978), a program that led to the foundation of the Primary Health Care Delivery Project (PHCDP) worldwide; it was further promoted in both the Millennium Development Goals (MDG) in 2000 and the Sustainable Development Goals (SDG) in 2015. Yet, with the above landmark inclusive health-care project, a number of human communities still suffer both social and economic deprivations preventing universal access to quality health-care services worldwide. Human communities, like rural, farming, and industrial settlements, socio-politically deprived populations, and violence-prone communities, are still inaccessible to quality health-care systems worldwide. In the United States of America (USA), racism prevents some human communities from accessing basic health-care services, and in many parts of Africa, where violence, poor political decisions, and poverty prevail, a large number of human communities are marginalized in accessing good quality health-care services. In India and Ecuador, inadequate infrastructure and poverty account for the marginalization of communities from accessing quality health-care services (Martin Eckhardt, Siw Carlfjord, Tomas Faresjö et al., 2019). Thus, communities deprived of accessing health-care systems are marginalized against quality health-care delivery. The effects are numerous, including high morbidity and mortality rates in marginalized communities, and the problem of carrying infections and health-care problems to favored communities.

Community marginalization against health-care services informs the social, political, and economic exclusions that prevent population residents in the affected communities from accessing quality health-care services. Such exclusion is often predicated on poor location of health-care infrastructure and inadequate provision of drugs to serve the population in the marginalized communities. Community exclusion in accessing quality health care can also be attributed to societal class structure, where people regarded as non-indigenes and low class in terms of economic and social features reside in specific communities that are deprived access to quality health care. The remoteness of the communities, characterized by poor communication and transportation access, can also lead to community marginalization against inclusive health-care delivery. People living in displaced communities as a result of violence, warfare, and natural disasters, like flooding, earthquakes, and the like, are often displaced from their original communities to be resettled elsewhere in places that lack the requisite quality health-care systems.

The above attracted attention to organize a colloquium involving humanity, social science, public health, pharmacy, nursing, health promotion, and any other health-related researchers having field-based data that can generate new discourses and build insights on the environment, economy, and health in marginal communities. The outcomes of the colloquium, supported by grants generated from the Group Research Linkage of the Alexander von Humboldt Foundation, Bonn, saw the selection of some of the presented papers at the colloquium as chapters in this editorial.

Beginning from the conceptual analysis of environment, economy, and health, access to health-care systems in some selected African marginal communities is critically examined. Drawing on ethnography conducted in Nigeria, South Africa, and Zimbabwe, the fifteen chapters published in this editorial discuss a wide range of issues concerning how environment and economy influence access to health-care systems in marginal societies. While most chapters in the editorial reflect area studies, they have far-reaching comparative effects on the larger context.

REFERENCES

Martin Eckhardt, Siw Carlfjord, Tomas Faresjö, et al. (2019). Universal Health Coverage in Marginalized Populations: A Qualitative Evaluation of a Health Reform Implementation in Rural Ecuador. *INQUIRY: The Journal of Health Care Organization, Provision, and Financing, Volume 56*: 1–10.

WHO. (1978). *Declaration of Alma-Ata. International Conference on Primary Health Care. September 6–12. Alma-Ata, USSR*. Geneva, World Health Organization.

Chapter 2

Beyond Aesthetics

Socio-Cultural Perspective and the Health Benefits of Selected Plants in Human Environment

Ọlálẹ́yẹ Samuel Káyọ̀dé and
Oyelàdé Olúfikáyọ̀ Kúnlé

INTRODUCTION

Environmental beautification is one of the primary responsibilities of every state in Nigeria particularly the urban cities, academic environments, and most especially, tertiary institutions and many of the well-planned estates. A very good example is the administration of former governor of Lagos State, Babatunde Fasola, which has continued to attract both local and international commendations for Lagos State. His tree planting, landscaping, and beautification projects were one of the best in his time. Today, however, "Fasola's flowers" have tremendously improved the aesthetics of Lagos as the Centre of Excellence and has also helped in checking the effects of global warming on the environment (Iwu & Gbodossou, 2000). Wherever there are activities like this, almost on a daily basis, one would see people clearing, cleaning, pruning, cutting, and watering gardens and parks, thus providing job opportunities for many especially not well-educated people in society. It is also an avenue for the professional horticulturists to have their trees and flowers sold.

Apart from the aesthetics, the greening initiative was a deliberate effort to alleviate the effect of climate change and protect the future of the environment. There is no doubt that global warming is real, and the effect of extreme weather conditions around the world has drawn a wakeup call. Nigeria is no exception to its negative impact. However, one may ask, aside from the beautification and aesthetic values of these plants, of what other benefits are the plants to the individuals and the society in general? The chapter is structured as follows: Theoretical Orientation, Plants in African Traditional Socio-Cultural Milieu, Plants: Beyond Aesthetic Nature of Human Environment, Major Findings, Further Discussion of Findings, Summary, and Conclusion and Recommendations.

THEORETICAL ORIENTATION: ECOLOGICAL MODEL

The Ecological Model is adopted to explain the crux of the study. The model refers to "the interaction between and interdependent of, factors within and across all levels of a health problem. It highlights people's interaction with their physical and socio-cultural environments" (See *Theory at a Glance: A Guide for Health Promotion and Practice*). Ecological models recognize multiple levels of influence on health behaviors. Among others are: the intrapersonal/individual factors, which influence behavior, such as knowledge, attitudes, beliefs, and personality; interpersonal factors, such as interactions with other people, which can provide social support or create barriers to interpersonal growth that promotes healthy behavior; institutional and organizational factors, including the rules, regulations, policies, and informal structures that constrain or promote healthy behaviors; community factors, such as formal or informal social norms that exist among individuals, groups, or organizations, which limit or enhance healthy behaviors; and public policy factors, including local, state, and federal policies and laws that regulate or support health actions and practices for disease prevention, including early detection, control, and management.

It is important to mention that the relevance of the ecological model to this study is established in the fact that the health behavior of many African people with regard to the application of environmental plants for health purposes is influenced by personal or private individual factors, such as awareness, attitudes, dogmas, and disposition. Again, whether social support or obstacles to relational progression, consequent to interpersonal features such as contacts with other individuals, enhance the health behavior of some people. Furthermore, institutional and organizational factors, community factors, and public policy factors, among others, do influence African health behavior with reference to the use of plants for healthy living. Hence, the majority of trees and plants with health benefits in the African context are still limited in their usage to aesthetic purpose.

PLANTS/TREES IN AFRICAN TRADITIONAL SOCIO-CULTURAL PERSPECTIVE

There are two basic understandings about the origin of plants: they are the evolution and the creation models. An account of the plants' evolution explains that plants evolved from the aboriginal green algae about four hundred million years ago; another holds that plants are as old as 475 million years, while some other scholars hold that all types of plants were created on the third day of creation (Roger, 2007; Kutamal et.al., 2015). All these suggest that the existence of plant is as old as humanity. However, for the purpose of this paper, we shall discuss plants and trees from the African traditional social and cultural perspective, particularly the significance attached to plants and trees in African tradition. The importance attached to trees and plants in African tradition cannot be dismissed with a wave of the hand. In fact, trees and plants to African people are as important as life itself. Hence, the question of why some plants and trees have a very high cultural value from African traditional socio-cultural milieu is worth examining. However, it is important to mention that the value trees and plants hold vary from culture to culture and person to person. The following, among others, explain some of these facts:

ECONOMIC BENEFITS OF TREES AND PLANTS

The economic importance of trees and plants cannot be overemphasized. In fact, whether directly or indirectly, plants and trees make copious contributions to the sustainability of livelihood and well-being of many rural people across the globe, especially through the provision of ecosystem-related services (Katerere et.al., 2009; Agwu, Anyanwu, Uduogu & Akinnagbe, 2008). This is particularly so in areas where the large rural population for their livelihood depends directly or indirectly on small-scale farming and natural resources (Katerere et al., 2009; Agwu, Anyanwu, Uduogu & Akinnagbe, 2008). An interviewee stated: "there are many things that we local people enjoy in having trees and plants around us. You know many of our people live on the products from the bush, firewood, coal, chewing stick, bamboo, etc. All these provide means of living for some of our people, in fact that is what I live on. Some do not engage in it as day-to-day business like I do, yet they do it as back-up" (Egin, 2020). Another stated, "some products are derived from certain trees that are real money, if one has them; cocoa, cashew, kola-nut, palm tree and so on. Our people plant such trees for survival, we deal so much with cocoa and palm trees in this area and people get rich from them"

(Adeoye, 2020). This is corroborated by the assertion that it is not strange to many traditional African regions to harvest products from trees and plants for economic purpose. They include but are not limited to fuel wood, chewing stick, oil bean, cashew, bitter kola, kola nut, oil palm fibre, bamboo, and timber, among others, especially for rural households (Onwubuya, Ogbonna and Ezeobiora, 2014). It has been scholarly established that rural households in Africa engage in the gathering and selling of forest tree leaves, fruits, seeds, and roots for income. In fact, it is held that they fall back on such activities for income and food most of the time so as to cope with crop failure, shortfalls in food supply, or any other form of financial emergency (Shackleton & Shackleton, 2004).

Trees as Windbreaker

It is meaningful that every house owner will want to protect his or her house from being blown away by the wind. This, over the years, has been experienced in many parts of Africa. Hence, the simple logic of planting trees that could serve as a windbreaker. In an interviewee's explanation: "On several occasions we have experienced wind blowing off building roofs such that serious damages are caused and to have them repaired is not easy, that has brought about the idea that trees be planted around houses to protect heavy wind against damages to our buildings" (Ojelabi, 2020). This is not illogical to the mind, especially in societies where rainstorms are usually experienced, and where this has claimed or threatened properties and lives of the people. Oje et al. (2020), in investigating the environmental benefits of trees in a changing climate, especially in Nigeria, considers windbreaking as one. It is important that public buildings like churches and mosques, as well as other important buildings in the community, are also protected from wind or rainstorms by trees planted in some African traditional settings.

Relaxation/Recreation and Location for Ethical Class

Africans acknowledge and appreciate the idea of recreation, such that after the day's work or even at moon time, they sit in front of the house under the tree for relaxation. They engage in games like *Ayò Ọ̀lọ́pọ́n*. At times, they crack jokes or engage in proverbs and aphorisms they consider relevant in the course of playing the game. In an interviewee's explanation: "Rest is sweet after labour is a popular saying. In those days, when our fathers came back from the farm, they would sit under the tree in front of the house to play, although that is not very much common today, but it still exists in many of our rural areas" (Oyediji, 2020). It is important to mention that such engagements under the tree have always enhanced the communal living and moral life of the people. They learn ethical lessons for everyday social life. This does not exclude the younger people. Most of the time, the older men and women engage the children in moonlight stories, tales, fables, and songs under a tree in the mood of relaxation to teach the children moral lessons that would be beneficial later in life. By these, many African cultural heritages are sustained; African ethics, philosophy, cultural values, and ways of life in general are taught as the younger generations ask questions for clarifications from the older people.

Plants and Trees for Fruit

Most economic among the sociocultural values of plants and trees in the African traditional setting is the food and fruits that some of them produce. Africans traditionally appreciate the benefits derived from fresh vegetables and fruits for healthy living. Hence, in some parts of Africa, vegetables and edible fruit trees are planted, not only in distant farm locations, but around the house, such that they are easily used when necessary. An interviewee attests to this when he asserted: "it is not only for domestic use that is a major business we embark upon here, and people all over the nation know us for it. It is our means of living" (Ogunmola, 2020). Fruit trees, such as mango, guava, orange, and cashew, are planted, and various vegetables are cultivated, not only for domestic use but also for commercial purpose.

Trees as Social and Cultural Symbolism

In Africa, particularly in southwestern Nigeria, some trees are appreciated for what they produce and for the cultural or social use of what they produce, perhaps in terms of fruits or what the society produces from such trees. For instance, kola nuts are used as a symbol of friendship and of welcome. Traditional prayers and ceremonies are usually started with the ceremonial breaking of a kola nut. An interviewee explained: "I am an Ibo woman, I got married to a Yoruba. You see, kola-nut to us in Ibo land is not just a seed, it has its significance in our culture. It is a symbol of friendliness and of welcome, it is life" (Alabi, 2020). Explaining this idea, Chudume et al. (2015) posits:

> To the Igbo, the kolanut is not just the small seed, in actual fact the seed is very bitter to taste. It is merely the non-juicy unattractive, reddish or yellowish small content of the pod of a tree called osisi oji (kolanut tree). The Oji tree does not grow to a great height. . . . Kolanut excels more in Igboland for socio-cultural significance compared to its value than in any other ethnic group in West Africa. . . . The fact is that the rites of presentation, blessing, breaking, and distribution of kola-nut in Igboland are much more solemn than we recognize. They

> symbolize a social and ritual bonding between the living on one hand, the living and the departed on the other. It is a ceremonial covenant of hosts and guests with benevolent ancestral spirits and deities in the presence of Ani, the Earth Deity (Chidume, Ossioma and Echem, 2015:51).

Palm trees also accord the same cultural status of togetherness and spirit of sharing, as palm wine derived from the tree serves traditional social purposes. In traditional prayer gatherings or ceremonies like marriage, libation is poured with palm wine, for instance. Hence, in African traditional settings, there are trees to which social and cultural symbolisms are attached.

Enhancement of Cooling Facility during the Hot Weather

Scientifically, the role of trees in human life in relation to climate change is worth mentioning. Climate scientists have always remarked that afforestation is a major component of climate-change adaptation. Among the functions of a forest is the offer of regular water availability by reducing the hot temperatures that could dry up water beneath the ground. It has been scholarly explained that by "evapotranspiration, trees rejuvenate atmospheric moisture, and contribute to rainfall at both local and in distant localities" (Ellison, Cindy, and Locatellie et al., 2017). Cooling is, therefore, undeniably fixed in the capability of trees to arrest and redeploy the sun's energy (Pokorný, Brom, Cermák et al., 2010). It is thus logical that trees are planted around the house such that during the dry season or hot weather conditions, they create cooling facilities for the inhabitants of such houses. This is not uncommon in African environments. In fact, in southwestern Nigeria, especially in the suburbs, people decide to sit outside under the tree for relief from the heat generated by the hot weather.

Trees Serve as Markers/Demarcation

Like they are used in many other African settlements, trees are used as landmarks or boundaries between one village and another, such that they carry a large amount of cultural value. In some cases, trees are used as demarcations between two farms. In this case, the ownership of the farmland is established between two individuals. It has been established that such trees over the years have enabled and facilitated solutions to the problem of land disputes, either between two individuals or families. Hence, the cultural values of trees in Africa as markers. Trees in many contemporary African settlements that have been used as markers at one point in time or the other in the past have over the years served as such with which areas are named. An interviewee said, "trees are usually used as landmark either for demarcation or identification of places, it is an age long idea that is why, particularly in some parts of Yoruba Land, for instance in Ibadan, we have areas being called Idi Obi (where a kola nut tree is located), Idi Ope (where a palm tree is located), Idi Osan (where an orange tree is located), and so on" (Oyejide, 2020). This is not different from the explanation of Borokini (2016) that trees in Africa, particularly in southwestern Nigeria, are used to name villages. Examples cited by Borokini include: Idi-Osan (where the citrus tree is located), Idi-Ayunre (where the *Albizia Odoratissima* tree is located), Idi-Ose (where the *Adansonia digitata* tree is located), Idi-Oro (where the *Irvingia gabonensis* tree is located), Idi-Ishin (where the *Blighia sapida* tree is located), Idi-Araba (where the *Ceiba petandra* tree is located), Idi-mangoro (where the *Mangifera indica* tree is located), etc. In view of this, the role trees play in the life of humanity particularly as markers is so crucial in the contemporary world, such that consciously or unconsciously, people refer to it on a daily basis in the society.

Attachment of Sacredness to Trees

In Africa, particularly in southwestern Nigeria, some trees hold immense cultural value and serve as sacred objects. Extant literature reveals that the veneration of sacred trees, groves, mountains, and rivers are very common among the Yoruba of southwestern Nigeria, to the extent that such is noted in virtually all communities (Borokini, 2016). The Ìrókò tree, Milicia explains, is one of the trees revered in southwestern Nigeria. It is used for various mystical purposes and traditional festivals. It is held across southwestern Nigeria and beyond that spirits known by different names, including Ọ̀rọ̀ or Olúwéré, live in the tree. It is also believed that witches also hold their meetings on top of the Iroko trees, particularly at night. It is important to mention that the Iroko tree is one among many trees that are held sacred among the Yoruba of southwestern Nigeria (Borokini, 2016).

THE PERSPECTIVE OF *IFÁ* DIVINATION ON PLANTS AND HUMAN ENVIRONMENT

The Yoruba are of the opinion that when the world was created through the indirect work of the divinities, it was the soil that was first created through Orunmila (Adeoye, 1985). Although some schools of thought believed it was Obatala (Salami, 2002), some viewed that it was Oduduwa (Idowu, 1982). Then plants were created in diverse kinds, beginning from the palm tree, which was the source of water for the divinities. The trees brought forth fruits of all kinds for the benefit of the living creatures. However, all these that Olodumare created, he put under the care of some special people before the creation of man. This is the reason Osanyin was placed in charge of plants and why he knows the secret of all the plants. He, however, transferred this knowledge to humans when man was eventually created. Osanyin, the tutelary spirit or doctor's divinity, as Bolaji Idowu (1982) calls the divinity, is believed to be the younger brother of Orunmila. However, there are other diverse claims about Osanyin. According to Adeoye, Osanyin and Orunmila were friends in heaven, but Osanyin later became Orunmila's slave as a result of inability to heed warning. *Ọ̀kànràn-Túrùpọ̀n* (Adeoye, 1985) attests to this fact where *Ifá* says:

Ifá kíkọ́ ni í múni mọfá	Learning Ifa makes one knows Ifa
Ọ̀nà ṣíṣì ni í múni mọ̀nà	Missing ones way makes one knows the way
Ọ̀nà táà á rìn rí	A road that one has not trekked before
Nií ṣeni ṣìbálá ṣìbolo	Is always puzzling
A dÍfá fún Ọ̀rúnmìlà	Casts divination for Orunmila
A kì fún Ọ̀sányìn Ewèlè	Divines for Osanyin Ewele
Lọ́jọ́ tí Olódùmarè dé Igbá sílẹ̀	On the day Olodumare covered a calabash
Tí Ọ̀rúnmìlà ní òun le kIfa	That Orunmila claimed that he would divine
Mọ oun tí n bẹ nínú igbá tí Olódùmarè dé kalẹ̀	To know what was in the calabash that Olodumare puts on the floor
Tí Ọ̀sanyìn ní dandan tàì dan	That Osanyin says compulsorily
Ibi tí Ọ̀rúnmìlà bá nlọ	Wherever Orunmila goes,
Ni Ọ̀sanyìn nrè	Is the place Osanyin will go
Tí Ifá npé òde ò dáa	That Ifa says that way is not okay
Ẹni a wífún kó gbọ́	He who is advised should abide
Ká sọ̀rọ̀fúnni ká gbà	If we are advised, we should take to it
Àwíìgbọ́, ògbe ọjọ́ kínní	Lack of taking to advise of that day
Ló sọ Ọ̀sanyìn dẹrú Ifá	Was what turned Osanyin to Ifa's slave.

Yet another one claimed that it was when both of them got to this world that Ọ̀sanyìn became his slave as a result of a war called *Ayéle* breaking out. Orunmila looked for Osanyin but could not get him. He consulted the oracle and was told Osanyin was in *okokòlọ́jọ́*, which could be interpreted as detention camp in our modern world. Ifá instructed that Orunmila should go around the slave market before Osanyin was sold into slavery. He went round and saw him at the Ejigbomekun market. He paid for his freedom and brought him home. Later he asked him to clear all the weeds in his compound, but Osanyin declined and told him the usefulness of those plants he had asked him to clear. Orunmila saw wisdom in what he said and gave him his freedom to be the head of herbalists till today. *Ògúndá Méjì* (Fasina Agboola, 1989) attests to this fact, where *Ifá* says:

Gbinrinbi iti, bi iti gbinrin,	Gbinrinbi iti, bi iti gbinrin,
A dIfá fun Orunmila	Cast divination for Orunmila
Nlora Osanyin lokoeru	He was going to buy Osanyin as a slave
Osanyin n be niigbekun	Osanyin was in a custody
Óún ráre lóko kòlọ́jọ́	He was suffering endlessly
Orunmila wa owo kan	Orunmila sourced for money
Baba lo re e ra Osanyin loko eru	He went to go and purchase Osanyin from the slave market
Orunmila mu Osanyin renu oko	Orunmila took Osanyin to his farm
Igba ti Osanyin de inu oko	When Osanyin got to the farm,
Igbe tantan l'Osanyin nke pe	He was shouting on top of his voice
Oko ti un o ro da	Where is the weed to be cleared
Gbinrinbiti	Gbinrinbiti
Eyi ewe aje	This leaf is for wealth
Gbinrinbiti	Gbinrinbiti
Oko ti un o ro da	Where is the weed to be cleared
Gbinrinbiti	Gbinrinbiti
Eyi ewe aiku	This one for longevity
Gbinrinbiti	*Gbinrinbiti*
Oko ti un o ro da	Where is the weed to be cleared
Gbinrinbiti	Gbinrinbiti

Another claim is of the opinion that Osanyin was fond of ridiculing Orunmila and his power. To this, Okanran-Turupon (Lijadu, 1965) says:

Ọ̀yígí lawo Ọ̀yígí	Oyigi is the priest of Oyigi
Ọ̀yígì lawo Ọ̀yígì	Oyigi is the priest of Oyigi
Ati dide l'a I mo agba ile si	Standing up is what elders are known for
A dIfá f'Osanyin	Casts divination for Osanyin
O nlo b'Orunmila leri	He was going to boast with Orunmila
Pe koseni to le yan oun m'ebo	That no one can count him as part of sacrificial materials.

Eventually, Orunmila indirectly included Osanyin as part of what he would use to offer sacrifice for Olofin. He begged Orunmila and voluntarily made himself his slave rather than for him to die. However, the long and short of the claims is that Osanyin was a slave to Orunmila. He was the one who taught him how to make use of plants as part of Orunmila's therapy for his clients because it was not part of his therapeutic mechanism. Rather, he made use of the Ebo-sacrifice only to solve all problems as attested to by *Ifá*, in *Ọ̀yẹ̀kú Ìká* (Ayo Salami, 2002) that:

Gúnnugún bà lórùlé	The vulture perches on top of a high wall
Ojú u rẹ̀ a tólé	Its gaze would cover the city
Ojú u rẹ̀ a tóko	Its gaze would cover the forest
A dIfá fún Ṣànìyàn	Cast divination for Saniyan
Ṣànìyàn tí nṣẹrú ìpín lọ́run	Saniyan the slave of destiny in heaven
Wọ́n ní ó rúbọ	He was asked to offer sacrifice
Oníkálukú ló ti yan ìpín	Everybody had chosen what he or she
Tí òun yió jẹ́ nínú ìyá ẹ̀	Would become during his or her sub-liminal stage
Nígbà tí nbọ̀ látòde ọ̀run . . .	When coming from the city of heaven . . .
. . . Ẹbọ lọ̀rúnmìlà mọ̀	. . . Orunmila is the one that knows no other thing than sacrifices
Gbogbo nkan tẹ́ẹ bá yàn tiò bá dáa	All those things which man chooses as destiny that is bad
Ọ̀rúnmìlà ni yió má a bá yín f'ẹbọ gbé e sójú ọ̀nà	It is he that would use sacrifice to mend it.

In contemporary times, it is very common in many of the *Ẹsẹ Ifá* to see that, in addition to the offering of sacrifice for the treatment of problems that emanated from divination, *Ifá* will prescribe *ewé Ifá*, herbs that are found in human environments for further treatment. However, this is always strictly according to the dictates of *Ifá.* Therefore, this indicates that the *Babalawo* cannot rely on his personal or previous experience to treat different clients with similar problems the same way.

BEYOND AESTHETIC: THE HEALTH BENEFITS OF SELECTED PLANTS IN HUMAN ENVIRONMENT

Plants are God-given gifts to human society. The importance of this gift can be seen in the activities and agitations of some countries in the desert areas that have no vegetation but desire it at all costs. These resulted in some of these countries spending huge sums of money in planting trees while some would go as far as creating artificial vegetation, because plants provide oxygen, without which there would be less fresh air to breathe for both animals and humans. This indicates that human survival depends greatly on plants. The importance of plants can also be seen in the provision of habitats for both animals and humans, most especially birds, which make their nests on branches of trees, and humans rely on plants to build their own houses (http://www.conserve-energy-future.com). Plants are the primary source on which both animals and humans rely for feeding and sustenance (http://www.worldwildlife.org). Well-planned and structured plants are beautiful to behold in many human environments, especially in urban city centres where the consciousness of planting is very high.

As earlier said, in the economic and social values of trees above, beyond using plants for several purposes, it is also relaxing for children to play games like *gbádígbádí*, *Bojúbojú*, and *Ọ̀bẹ̀ké*, and it provides a place to learn different songs. A good example of such a song is:

Làbẹ̀ igí órombò	Under the orange tree
Nìbẹ̀ la gbé nṣerewa	There we stay to play
Inu wa dùn,	We are happy
Ara wá yà	We are healthy
Làbè igí órombò.	Under the orange tree

Trees are also a good location for local musicians to practice their new songs. However, besides all the usefulness mentioned above, all these plants are also good and are used for medicinal purposes for humans to live healthy lives. Therefore, as explained from the biblical perspective in Ezekiel 12:47, plants were created for two major reasons: the fruits for eating and the roots for healing, which is the main reason for this paper: that is, to look at the purpose of plants beyond using them for the decoration of homes and environment. As a result, we shall look at medicinal values of some common plants in the human environment.

For instance, *polyalthia longifolia*, which belongs to the family of *Annonaceae*, and is known for its various names, is one of such plants that are common in the human environment for its decorative and beatification properties. It is commonly called ashoka, deodari in Hindi, ulkatah, kastadaru in Sanskrit, debdaru in Bengali, and unboi in Assamese (Katkar, Suthar, and Chauhan, 2010). It is also known as the masquerade tree, and the Yoruba call it Igi Ìgunnukó because of its striking resemblance to the Ìgunnukó masquerades in Badagry area of Lagos and Ogun states. It is one of the trees that are commonly used in the big cities and individual modern houses for beautification and decorative functions. In India, it is known for its spiritual qualities, as well as for its many health benefits to the body. The tree is dedicated to the love god, Karma, and the name is interpreted to mean 'no grief' in Sanskrit. Its medicinal values include treating menstrual problems in women, dysmenorrhea, abdominal pain, and uterine spasms. It also helps in the treatment of acne, improves intellect, and prevents internal bleeding, diarrhea, kidney stones, and asthma (DrxHina Firdous, 2019). The leaf of the tree is very good for the treatment of high blood pressure. The plant is also good for the treatment of septic infections, coughing, and cancers. The bark is useful in fever, while the root and seeds are very good for skin treatment (Adebayo Oluwole, 2020).

Hog plum-spondias mombin, which belongs to the family *Anacardiacae*, is another plant that is found in the rainforest of the Yoruba. It is called Ìyeyè in Yoruba and commonly used for living fences, tents for ceremonies, farmland demarcation, and shelter by artisans; it is planted to provide shade for relaxation at the same time as to play indoor games as a result of its ability to germinate easily. The fruits are edible, particularly for children. The wood is used for carving images and can sometimes be used as firewood for cooking. Research has shown that the fruit is a means of alleviating thirst. The ripe fruits are eaten out of hand or stewed with sugar. The extracted juice is used to prepare ice cream, cool beverages, and jelly in Costa Rica and Brazil. It is used in Panama, Peru, and Mexico in fairly large quantities as jams because it is very high in vitamin C, vitamin B1, iron, and calcium (Bose Akinsola, 2015). The fruits can also be used to produce wine, vinegar, and other drinks in many countries of the world like Mexico and Guatemala, where the three can be grown (Ayoka, Akomolafe, Akinsomisoye and Ukponmwan, 2008).

Beyond the usage of the Hog plum plant for the above-mentioned functions, the medicinal values are enormous. Crushed leaves or the infusion of hog plum can be used to reduce or relieve pain, sedate or calm, treat coughs, reduce fevers, and stop convulsions. It can also be used to aid digestion, stimulate the womb, kill parasites, treat mouth sores and infections, and treat inflammation. According to Jumoke, one herbal seller at the Òjé market affirmed that a tea made from the flowers and leaves is good for stomachache, vomiting, and eye and throat infections. She also claimed the bark can be prepared into a concoction and used to treat diarrhea and dysentery, relieve pain, treat hemorrhoids, stop bleeding, and treat skin disorders like eczema, dermatitis, boils, rashes, itches, leprosy, etc. The leaves and the bark of the tree can also be used also to eliminate parasites, to induce labour or abortion, and as a contraceptive (Jumoke Adenrele). Another informant is of the opinion that the bark, when combined with the leaf of Àtòrìn, Àrìndan, Ìyèré, and Atare, can be used to prepare a delicious soup to cure pile (Olabanle Olutayo). Again, if the root is made into concoctions, it can be used to treat vaginal infections, gonorrhea, and other venereal diseases. It is also good for diarrhea (Foluso Ogunleye).

Another good and beneficial plant in the human environment is *epimedium*, or goat weed, commonly called Imi Esu in Yoruba society. Though it is not planted for the purpose of beautification, it is beautiful to behold wherever it is found because of its flowers. One can almost say it is the most common plant found growing around human environment, bushes, and farms. It is a popular plant known to everyone without the knowledge of its medicinal values. Goat weed is a good remedy for many ailments in human society. According to Wilson (Debra Rose Wilson, 2017), goat weed is a form of alternative medicine for the treatment of hay fever, atherosclerosis, nerve pain, fatigue, osteoporosis, and erectile dysfunction.

In Yoruba society, too, the goat weed plant is used for similar purposes mentioned above. However, in addition to that, other health benefits of the plant according to Adeleye (2020), include fertility problems in women, weight loss, and ulcer treatment. It's a natural fertilizer for the soil. It is also good for abdominal and back pain, relief for headache and menstrual pain, and relief for cough and fever in children. It is an excellent remedy for poisonous bites/stings and an antidote against evil spells. Odunlofin (2020) is of the opinion that the plant can also be used to make a spiritual soap called Àwúre for bathing to receive favour from people. To this effect, its name is changed to Ṛ́érínkòmí while harvesting it solely for that purpose. He said further that the plant can also be used for a sexual remedy in men by processing and taking the juice of the plant; it cures urinary tract infections and is good for taking care of nose bleeds with just a drop of the juice in the nostrils and lying with the head up for a few minutes.

Hibiscus *sabdariffa* is another plant used in the beautification of the human environment, most especially schools, churches, and individual homes. However, research has shown that many health benefits can be derived from this plant. These benefits range from a tea made from the plant in boiling water that can lower blood pressure, fight bacteria, and aid weight loss (Rachael Link, 2017). The fleshy red calyx is used in the preparation of jams, jellies, and cold and warm teas and drinks. It is also good as a chemo preventive agent against tumor promotion in laboratory and animal studies. It is used in preventing renal stone formation, along with its respiratory and sedative effects. It can be used as a laxative, as well as a sperm buster, as viewed by Taiwo Ojo (2020).

Again, jatropha leaves—or the Làpálàpá plant—was used in the olden days to demarcate boundaries and make fences against animal disturbances. However, the usefulness of làpálàpá, as it is commonly called in Yoruba society, health-wise cannot be quantified as it has been popularly used to cure various diseases for ages. There are basically two types of this plant in Yoruba land; Làpálàpá pupa and làpálàpá funfun. The two are used for different purposes and can be sometimes mixed together to achieve a better result. From the leaves of jatropha to its root, the entire plant can be combined into the medicine therapy, physically and spiritually. Sometimes it can be combined with other medicinal herbs to get a better result.

Several methods can be used to process the jatropha leaves for use for the body's health. These range from eating it raw, cooking it like a vegetable, grinding it into powder that the Yoruba call àgúnmu or àgúnjẹ, depending on the locality, to grinding it raw—àlọ̀jẹ—and drinking it directly, or blending and filtering its essence to be taken to cure scars on the skin of the body skin (Ajayi Ageje, 2020). Sometimes it can be heated to be spread on the surface of a wound after using the sap to stop the bleeding of a fresh wound. Apart from curing the skin's blisters and scratches, as explained above, due to its essential protein and vitamins that regenerate and revitalize the skin cells' recovery, it can also be used for rheumatism as a result of its rich flavonoid, anti-oxide, protein, calcium, and potassium. For this purpose, the leaves are either boiled for drinking or stewed. The jatropha plant can also be used for defecation smoothing, skin problems, fever, jẹ̀díjẹ̀dí-dysentery, relief of infection, vitality for men, vaginal discharge, Ẹ̀dà-dripping of sperm in women, ear infection, cervical cancer, and antibiotics against venereal diseases (Ajayi Ageje, 2020).

Delonixregia belongs to the family of *Fabaceae* with the common name of *Gulmohar*. It is believed to have originated from Madagascar, and from there it spread to every other part of the world where it can be found today. It is called fire tree, the flambouyant/flanboyant tree, the flame tree gold mohn, the peacock flower, and the royal poinciana in English. In Hindi and Hawaii, it is known as Gulmohar. In Arab, it is called Goldmore, while in Bengali it is known as Krishachura. French people call it Flamboyan, while the Chinese call it Feng huang hua, or Hong hua ying, and the Yoruba called it Ṣẹkẹṣẹkẹ, possibly because of the sound the pod containing the seeds makes when shaking (Godofredo U. Stuart Jr., 2016). Delonixregia is a large tree with a fast-growing rate. It has fanlike leaves, beautiful red flowers, and green flat fruit when it is young. When matured, it turns black with hard, smooth, and well-arranged seeds in the pod. It is a fast-growing tree that provides shade for people to rest under. It is a windbreaker and a shelter for animals.

However, because of its aggressive root system, it is a good tree to help control soil erosion.

Economically, its wood is good for agricultural implements and handles for carpentry tools, etc. The seeds are processed for the fatty oil known as the pangam or karanga oil of commerce that is used in the tanning industry, in soap making, and in the pharmaceutical industry. Medicinally, the seed, when processed, purifies and enriches the blood and treats inflammation, "earache," and chest complaints (http://greencleanguide.com). Also, a collection of the seeds, together with the pod, can be burned together and used to care for dizziness—Òyì ojú (Alimot Motunrayo, 2020).

Studies also show that *Delonixregia* is antibacterial, anti-inflammatory, with flowers constituents/phenols and flavonoids, hepatoprotective/cytotoxic, antimicrobial, antidiarrheal, seed mucilage/tablet binder, wound healing/flowers, antidiabetic/leaves, hepatoprotective/anticancer/antioxidant, mercury absorption/anticancer/antioxidant, in vitro cytotoxic activity/flowers/cancer cell lines, antibacterial/root bark, an tnociceptive/cytotoxic/leaves, diuretic/flowers and corrosion inhibitor/aluminum, etc. (Godofredo U. Stuart Jr., 2016).

CONCLUSION

Olodumare the Creator in his infinite mercy created nature and made us the lord over it, and nature, in turn, has given us more than enough to care for our very selves. However, through man's negligence, uncaring attitude, indolence, and laziness, human beings have been plunged into self-created problems. As a result, humans began to look for God afar off whereas he is near—nearer, indeed, than our iṣan ọrùn—neck nerves. The Almighty created nature for human use, and man has neglected it. Man does not understand nature, much less God as the father. Olodumare ordered elemental beings to nourish and take care of these plants on behalf of man. They often teach humans how to make the best use of the plants for the good and benefit of man. They also plan ahead of any epidemic outbreak by planting herbs that would be used to take care of such an outbreak. However, through man's silly ways, man regarded these elemental beings as gods and began to worship them, without the knowledge that the elemental beings, too, knew the only person worthy of worship is the Almighty God, the Creator of the heavens and earth. They therefore stopped their services by not teaching humans the use of these herbs any longer, except those who regarded them as the servants of Olodumare. Thus, neglecting and abandoning man to his problem and lack of understanding, Olodumare is not stupid by creating nature before man. He knows from his infinite power that man will need all these things, and that is the reason he created them before man. If man, therefore, wakes up to his responsibility and makes nature his friend again, man shall have less problem on this mother earth, for truly the earth is the mother earth to man.

REFERENCES

Achebe, C. (2012). *There was a country: A personal history of Biafra*. London: Penguin Press.

Adeleye Taiwo, professional herbal seller/practitioner, Personal Interview, Bode Market, Ibadan, 11/12/2020.

Adeoye, C. L. (1985). *Igbagbo ati Esin Yoruba.* Ibadan: Evans Brothers (Nigeria Publishers) Limited.

Agabje-Williams, B. (2005). Clothed Ritual Trees: An Insight into Yoruba Religious Thought. In Renne, E. & Agabje-Williams, B. (eds.), *Yoruba Religious Textiles: Essays in Honour of Cornelius Oyeleke Adepedgba*. Ibadan: Book Builders

Agboola, Fasina. (1989). *Ojulowo Oriki Ifa, Apa Kinni*. Lagos: Project Publication Limited.

Agwu, A. E., Anyanwu, A. C., Uduogu, T. O., & Akinnagbe, O. A. (2008). The contributions of nait-nusho programme to poverty alleviation in Enugu North Agricultural Zone, Enugu State, Nigeria. *Journal of Tropical Agriculture, Food, Environment and Extension* 7(2): 129–38.

Ajayi Ageje, Ifa priest/herbalist-Sawosesegun, Telephone Interview, Ijelu Ekiti, 10/26/2020.

Akinsola, Bose (2015). *The health benefit of hog Plum*, http://1.bp.blogspot.com. Retrieved on 10/24/2020.

Alimot Motunrayo, herbs seller, Personal Interview, Ajibode, Ibadan, 11/23/2020.

Ayoka, A. O., Akomolafe, R. O., Akinsomisoye, O. S., and Ukponmwan, O. E. (2008). Medicinal and Economic Value of Spondias Mombin, *African Journal of Biomedical Research*, 11(2): 129–36.

Borokini, T. I. (2016). *Sanctuary of the Spirits: Okwu-muo, Ori Oke and 'Mammy Water' in the Veneration of Sacred Natural Sites in Southern Nigeria.* Plant Genetic Resources Unit, National Centre for Genetic Resources and Biotechnology (NACGRAB). Moor Plantation, Ibadan, Nigeria.

Chidume, C. G., Ossioma, U. S., Echem, S. O. (2015). The Symbolism of Kolanut in Igbo Cosmology: A Re-Examination. *International Journal of Research in Humanities and Social Studies*, 2(8): 51–56.

DrxHina Firdous (2019). *Benefits of Ashoka Tree and Its Side Effects.* http://www .lybrate.com.

Ellison, D., Cindy, E. M., Locatellie, B., Sheil, D., Cohen, J., Murdiyarso, D., Gutierrez, V., van Noordwijk, M., Creed, I. F., Pokorny, J., Gaveau, D., Spracklen, D. V., Tobella, A. B., Ilstedt, U., Teuling, A. J., Gebrehiwot, G. S., Sands, D. C., Muyst, B., Verbist, B., Springgay, E., Sugandi, Y., Sullivan, C. A. (2017). Trees, forests and water: Cool insights for a hot world. *Global Environmental Change*, 43:51–61.

Foluso Ogunleye, professional herbalist, Personal Interview through Phone, Itapa Ekiti, Ekiti State, 10/30/2020.

Fuwape, J. A. (2003). Role of forests in poverty alleviation and sustainable development in West Africa. http://www.fao.org/docrep/ARTICLE/WFC/XII/0123-A2.HTM.

Idowu, Bolaji. (1982). *Olodumare God in Yoruba Belief.* Lagos: Longman Nigeria Limited.

Iwu, M. M., and Gbodossou, E. (2000). The role of traditional medicine. *Lancet*, 356, doi.10.1016/S0140-6736 (00)91989–5.

Jumoke Adenrele, herbs seller, Oje Market, Ibadan, Personal Interview, 10/22/2020.

Katerere, Y., Minang, P., and Vanhanen, H. (2009). *Making Sub-Saharan African forests work for people and nature, Policy approaches in a changing global environment.* Nairobi, Kenya, World Agroforestry Centre.

Katkar, K. V., Suthar, A. C., and Chauhan, V. S. (2010). *The Chemistry, Pharmacologic, and Therapeutic Applications of* Polyalthia Longifolia, www.ncbi.nlm.nih.gov. Retrieved on 10/21/2020.

Kutama1, A. S., Dangora, I. I., Aisha, W., Auyo, M. I., Sharif, U., Umma, M., and Hassan, K. Y. (2015). An overview of plant resources and their economic uses in Nigeria. *Global Advanced Research Journal of Agricultural Science*, 4(2): 42–67, Available online http://garj.org/garjas/index.htm.

Lijadu, E. A. (1965). *Ifa Mimo Alabalase.* Ado Ekiti: United Star Printers Ltd, 21.

Link, Rachael (2017). Eight Benefits of Hibiscus Tea, https://www.healthline.com.

N.a., 2020, Fifteen Benefits of Jatropha Leaves (Anu Agro Farm Limited), https://m.facebook.com, retrieved from internet on 11/23/2020.

Odunlofin Thomas, traditional birth attendant, Telephone Interview, Itapa Ekiti, 10/10/2020.

Ojeh, V. N., Philip-Humshie, A., Garba, H. A., Naabil, E., Obiano, E. C., Boyitie, O. P., and Boyiga, K. K. (2020). The Environmental Benefits of Trees in a Changing Climate: A Nigerian Experience. *Journal of Scientific Research & Reports* 26(6): 59–75.

Olabanle Olutayo, civil servant/herbalist, Personal Interview, Oranyan Area, Ibadan, 10/22/2020.

Oluwole, Adebayo. (2020). *Masquerade Tree (Polyalthia Longifolia): The False Ashoka*, positivepsychology.org.ng, retrieved 11/23/2020.

Onwubuya, E. A., Ogbonna, O. I., and Ezeobiora, O. C. (2013). Conservation of forest resources by rural farmers in Anambra State, Nigeria. *Journal of Agricultural Extension* 18(2). http://dx.doi.org/10.4314/jae.v18i2.18

Pokorný, J., Brom, J., Cermák, J., and Hesslerová, P. (2010). Solar energy dissipation andTemperature control by water and plants. *Int. J. Water*, 5: 311–36. DOI: 10.1504/IJW.2010.038726.

Puskar, E. (2018). *Economic Importance of Delonixregia*, http://greencleanguide.com. Retrieved 24/11/2020.

Roger, P. (2007). *The Origin of Plants.* Oxford: Oxford University Press, 246.

Salami, Ayo. (2002). *Ifa: A Complete Divination.* Lagos: NIDD Publishing and Printing Limited, 85. http://www.conserve-energy-future.com/carbon-sinks.php, retrieved on 11/12/2020.

Shackleton, C., and Shackleton, S. (2004). The importance of non-timber forest products in rural livelihood security and as safety nets: A review of evidence from South Africa. *South African Journal of Science*, 100: 658–64.

Stuart Jr., Godofredo U. (2016). *Philippine Medicinal Plants Flamboyant Tree.* https://stuartXchange.org, retrieved on 11/22/2020.

Taiwo Ojo, herbalist, oral interview, Ago Tailor Area, Ibadan, 10/23/2020.

Wilson, Debra Rose (2017). *What's to know about horny goat weed?* http://www.medicalnewstoday.com, retrieved on 10/30/2020.

NOTE

Permissions were granted to reprint the verbatim quotations in this report and the names are anonymized.

Chapter 3

Revitalization of Herbal Medicine

A Challenge to Orthodox Medicine

Ayotunde Olayori Oguntade

INTRODUCTION

Man has always been confronted with the need to live a healthy life. If he will be successful and have the opportunity to eat the fruit of his labor, he must be healthy. It is a popular saying in the African setting that "health is wealth." According to African belief, some forces usually militate against the health of the man; these may be spiritual or physical. In most cases, they believe that events do not just take place. Thus, events, and in this case illnesses, are mostly interpreted in the framework of a magic or religious background (Oosthuisen, 1968, p. 87). It should be noted that they also believe that some ailments are a result of natural causes, bad habits, or self-inflicted problems. To subdue these forces, many approaches have been invented by African traditionalists; one of these is called herbal medicine. Herbal medicine is different from orthodox medicine in two ways. First, it makes use of plant roots, leaves, flowers, and seeds and retains its naturality. This is unlike orthodox medicine, which has to pass through a chemical process (Ogunyale, 2009). Before the advent of civilization in most cases, herbal medicine was a combination of herbs and magic substances or rituals. The reason for this is connected to the world milieu of Africans, who view almost every event from a spiritual perspective without a link to scientific knowledge or discovery. On the other hand, the orthodox medicine practitioners examine health challenges from a scientific perspective without consideration to the possibility of spiritual factors. There should be a balance between these two extremes. Secondly, herbal medicine is different from orthodox medicine because in most cases it is prepared and administered by indigenous medical practitioners who have often relied on personal experiences and consultations with the more experienced traditionalists.

Until fairly recently, herbal medicine had been criticized and condemned by Westerners. They believed that herbal medicine was substandard because they did not pass laboratory tests, whereas Africans relied on tested and proven experiences. It was also condemned because of the magic substances and rituals that are usually attached to the production and application of African medications. They often label "their treatments witchcraft" (Falk, 1997, p. 446). To them, it is unreasonable to believe that the unseen natural world could bring healing. Despite these criticisms and condemnations, it is a known fact that "much of what was known about orthodox medicine in its early days came from traditional medicine. Pharmacology developed from herbalism and many drugs are still derived from plants" (Ajayi, 2009).

In recent times, there has been a revitalization of herbal medicine. It is not an overstatement to note that in this contemporary time, there is keen competition between orthodox medicine and herbal medicine. Herbal medicine is becoming more popular and acceptable to Africans. Consequently, herbal medicine poses a challenge to orthodox medicine. This calls for a reexamination of the former disposition to African medicine for a possible collaboration between African orthodox medicine practitioners and their counterparts of herbal medicine practitioners. This collaboration will help greatly in developing a health system that suits the African cultural context.

HERBAL MEDICINE IN RETROSPECT

The art and science of restoring and preserving health have existed since time immemorial (Nabofa, 1993). In Africa, the oral tradition has it that medicine emanated from religion. This is because it came directly from a supreme deity and operated through a tutelary divinity or spirits (Idowu, 1973, p. 199). Among the Yoruba, the tutelary divinity of medicine is *Osanyin*, believed to be the younger brother of *Orunmila*, the divine consultant about human destiny (Idowu, 1973, p. 200). Therefore, in Africa, the sick consulted their priest for healing. This is because therapy was regarded as "the possession of a Divine Healer who dispensed it through the agency of a priest" (Idowu, 1973).

In some instances, in the African traditional setting, magic and medicine were combined. In such instances, the collection of ingredients and application of medicine was accompanied by some form of ritual. Furthermore, the mention of the invocation of ancestors in connection with the practice of medicine was a common feature in the practice of medicine in many parts of Africa. It was an accepted practice that apart from God and/or the divinity, the ancestors who first practiced the medicine must be given due honor. It was believed that this would make the medicine to be efficacious (Idowu, 1973, p. 200). Traditional doctors in Africa often claimed that they were taught medicine by divinities or in dreams, in trances, or during meetings with spirits in forests (Idowu, 1973, p. 200). Corroborating this argument, Mrs. M.A. Ogunyale said that her late husband, though the son of an herbalist, also got the inspiration for herbal medicine from his dreams, and that her husband, being a psychologist, established the awareness that herbal medicine is more effective for Africans than is orthodox medicine through his studies.

It is insightful to point out that ritual was important, because to them unconsecrated medicine had no meaning. That is why divine and ancestral sanctions were considered necessary before and during the preparation and application of medicine (Ogunyale, 2009). The combination of magic or ritual with herbs was also important because it was believed that the illness was a physical manifestation of spiritual decay (Nadel, 1954, p. 73). Therefore, treating the illness, in the indigenous view, meant conjuring up energy that would repair the spiritual state so that the spiritual healing would be translated into physical healing (Nadel, 1954, p. 73). Because of this, an attempt would be made to know the historical background of the patient and the reason for the physical illness (this is the traditional way of diagnosing illness). After obtaining this knowledge, the consultant would move to the next stage, which has to do with getting the plants, the roots, and the leaves (Nadel, 1954, p. 74). Most of these medicine plants fall into the corridor of food therapy (Babalola, 2006, p. 184). It is common knowledge that orthodox medicine professionals have also been emphasizing the importance of eating a balanced diet as a strategy for preventing illness and also for curative purposes.

It should, therefore, be pointed out that although traditional practitioners did not make use of modern diagnostic equipment in ascertaining causations, there were indigenous methods for diagnosis. These include divination, "traditional histology," invocation of supernatural forces, water or oil gazing, visual observation of the patients' urine, tongue, palms, excreta, and skin, and feeling or smelling the patients' noses and ears (Osunwole, 1993). This was unlike orthodox doctors, who make use of medical apparatus such as stethoscopes, which enable them to listen to the beating of the heart and sounds of breathing. They also carry out some laboratory examinations of patients' urine, excreta, or blood (Weikang, 1985, p. 1). The herbal medicine practitioners at that time neither had knowledge nor access to scientific equipment, but they made use of the ones revealed to them through instinct and divinities. It is then obvious that in the African traditional setting, the effectiveness of medicine depends on four things: traditional diagnosis, consultation with divinities and ancestors, materials (herbs), and incantation.

It should also be added that medicine was more often than not prescribed with the instruction that it must be used at stated times. It must also be used under certain conditions, accompanied by certain prescribed gestures (which may be repetitive), and given with incantations. Hence, from the point of view of the patient, it was difficult to know whether it was medicine or the accompanying ceremonies or both that effected the cure (Idowu, 1973, p. 202). Thus, in hindsight, the lack of laboratory procedures was a major disadvantage of herbal medicine. It may also not be preserved or stored for a long time (Oyebisi, 2009); aside from this, its side effects could not be ascertained (Nihinlola, 2009). Furthermore, as a result of the lack of laboratory procedures, the measurement of dosage was by chance, not by scientific calculation. Thereby, the patient had the risk of taking an overdose or an underdose (Oyekan, 2009). According to all orthodox practitioners' respondents, the probability of overdose is higher than underdose. Ajayi (2009) writes in this direction thus:

> What then is the difference between modern-day medicines and traditional medications? Simply put, when you take herbal medicine, you are taking a whole egg with its shell, the white and the yolk when it is only the yolk inside that is beneficial. In modern medicine, the shell and the white would have been carefully separated by technological processes leaving the yolk which is the active ingredient. There is no such luxury as traditional herbal medicine you take.

In the view of traditional African medicine practitioners, the issue of dosage has been discovered through several years of practice. Therefore, the nature and intensity of the sickness will determine the dosage to be used. However, it should not be considered to be out of place that there is the need for herbal medicine to undergo laboratory procedures because all the articles in the herbs may not be needful for the healing. The next section puts into consideration efforts that have been made to modernize or renew herbal medicine.

REVITALIZATION OF HERBAL MEDICINE

There is an ongoing revival of herbal medicine. This is obvious in so many ways. First, there is a transformation in the nomenclature; for example, the titles *herbalist*, *juju man*, or *witch doctor* have now changed to *doctor*. Formerly, they were addressed in these ways for diverse reasons. They were addressed this way because of various biases of writers, especially European writers. Also, the ways practitioners of the art professed their art and the variability of culture, which invariably gives credence to the existence of the art, made them be addressed as herbalists or witch doctors (Owumi, 1993).

Today, however, there is an ongoing reformation of the profession of the art. Likewise, African traditional medicine is now known as "trado-herbal medicine." Secondly, an effort is also being made to drastically reduce some of the ancient traditional mystical elements of herbal medicine. Thirdly, the National Agency for Food and Drug Administration and Control (NAFDAC) is now approving some of these herbal medicines. It is also receiving high public awareness through the media, nationally and internationally. Some of these herbal medicine clinics have websites on the internet.

Thus, it is now becoming more obvious that there are two types of herbalists in African religions. There are pure herbalists and diviner herbalists. The pure herbalist does not combine herbal remedies with divination and the mystical powers of the spirit world. Gehman (1989, 77), citing Daidanson, argues that: "to say that there were no pure herbalists is not true. Sometimes people were told to collect certain herbs, use them and be healed. But if that same herbalist/diviner required that person to return the next day with a hen or an egg that showed a religious element was involved." Supporting this position, Ogunyale (2009) said that in their traditional clinic, they do not practice palm reading, divination, and ritual.

There are three kinds of activities in African religion. There are activities that are not committed to religious beliefs, though this may be hard to find in traditional African culture. There are also activities that are religiously committed and activities that are mixed. Some herbal specialists freely give herbal medicines without any religious connotations, while others give the same herbs for the same illness because of religious/spiritual reasons (Gehman, 1989, pp. 77–78). For example, the Ogunyale traditional clinic does not recommend ritual, but it does require laboratory results and in some cases a doctor's report (Ogunyale, 2009). This is the greater reason why African drugs are now being prepared in a modern way. Herbal medicine now comes out in capsules, tablets, and liquid-like orthodox medicine. This causes it to compete with orthodox medicine.

The traditional system of thought in contemporary times has clearly shown that diseases can occur naturally in the course of human interaction with the physical environment. For example, there is the belief that diseases can occur naturally as a result of germs or worms. These may reside in the stomach, blood, skin, or any other part of the body (Osunwole, 1993). This new understanding is being promoted in various advertisements in the media sponsored by trado-herbal medicine practitioners. Thus, the emphasis on illness is now on natural causes than on spiritual attack.

CHALLENGES OF HERBAL MEDICINE TO ORTHODOX MEDICINE

There is no gainsaying in pointing out that the revitalization of herbal medicine is a challenge to orthodox medicine. Herbal medicine poses many challenges to orthodox medicine. This section examines these challenges.

First, herbal medicine has continued to appeal to the people despite the availability of orthodox medicine. In view of this, there is low patronage of orthodox medicine, especially in local areas. This implies that it is a challenge for orthodox practitioners to reexamine their positions on herbal medicine. Babalola (2006, p. 185) observes that there are cases when modern therapy is unable to provide the solution and the patient is advised to look for the solution via alternative therapy (that is, herbal medicine).

Second, as a result of its acceptability by the public, orthodox medicine is gradually becoming an alternative to herbal medicine. According to Oguntade (2009), a nurse at State Hospital Oyo, herbal medicine complicates the service of orthodox practitioners. This is because some patients after patronizing herbal medicine practitioners would come for orthodox treatment. She cited an example of a case of prolonged labour due to the use of a herbal medical ring. She asserts that this has always created a scenario of confusion. This example given by Oguntade may not be commendable, but from this, we can deduce that there is a gradual shift in the order of preference between orthodox medicine and herbal medicine.

Third, African medicine is gradually gaining international recognition. African herbal medicines are now being exported and refined and brought back for sale. Most of our needs, therefore, are managed through the repackaging of herbal medicine. Moreover, the World Health Organization (WHO) is now gradually recognizing some herbal medicines. For instance, China is one of the richest countries in the world in terms of herbal medicine. India is also making headway in this regard. Therefore, there is a challenge to continue to research African traditional medicine. This has started, but it should be intensified. Researchers and scholars are now doing important work on herbal medicine. There is now cross-fertilization of knowledge between African traditional medicine and modern medicine (Babalola, 2006, p. 185). For example, there is provision for the training of traditional birth attendants on how to conduct a safe delivery. They are trained on what to use to cut the cord, to have a clean environment for delivery, and not to allow the pregnant woman to bear down on a cervix that is not fully dilated (Oguntade, 2009). It should be noted that most herbal medicine practitioners have little to no knowledge of human anatomy and what constitutes the psycho-chemistry of the human body. Consequently, they do not understand fully the causes of most ailments (Adesina, 2009). Therefore, a forum or fora for training should be encouraged. This is because it is certain that some people will continue to patronize herbal medicine practitioners.

CONCLUSION

This chapter has discussed the reawakening of herbal medicine in contemporary times. It has revealed that herbal medicine is receiving high patronage and demand. Therefore, it is posing a great challenge to orthodox medicine practitioners to reconsider their positions on herbal medicine. Peter Falk observes that "in recent years medical authorities are recognizing the validity of many African cures through the use of native herbs. Serious study of specific remedies is being made. Late as this recognition is, it is valuable for the future development of more natural cures" (Falk, 1997, p. 450).

It has been discovered that despite civilization, herbal medicine is still thriving. In light of this, it is obvious that herbal medicine cannot be eradicated from Africa. Therefore, there is a need to work on its improvement, especially in the areas of refinement and removal of African traditional mystical elements. To achieve these, there is a need for cross-fertilization of knowledge between the orthodox practitioners and herbal practitioners. There is also the need for the government to seek its improvement and development, like in the cases of China and India, which have been cited.

REFERENCES

Ajayi, Ben. (2009). Modern Medicine and Traditional Medicine. *Nigerian Tribune*, May 7.

Babalola, E .O. (2006). The Impact of African Magic and Medicine on the Growth and Development of Modern Nigeria: The Yoruba Experience. In Raji, R. A. et al. (eds.). *Religion, Governance and Development in the 21st Century.* Ibadan, Macmillan, 27–52.

Falk, Peter (1997). *The Growth of the Church in Africa.* ACTS.

Gehman, R. J. (1989). *African Traditional Religion in Biblical Perspective.* Kesho Publications.

Idowu, E. B. (1973). *African Traditional Religion.* Lagos, SCM Press, Ltd.

———. "Religion, Magic and Medicine—with Special Reference to Africa," ORITA: Ibadan, *Journal of Religious Studies*, 1(2).

Nabofa, M. Y. (1993). Faith/Spiritual Healers as Alternative Therapeutics: Successes and Failure. In Oke, E.A. and Owumi, B.E. (Eds). *Readings in medical sociology.* Lagos, RMDS Publisher, 58–67.

Nadel, S. F. (1954). *Nupe Religion.* Routledge & Kegan Paul, Ltd.

Oosthuisen, G. C. (1968). *Post-Christianity in Africa.* Hurst.

Osunwole, S. A. (1993). Diseases diagnosis and etiology as system of thought. In Oke, E.A. and Owumi, B.E. (eds). *Readings in Medical Sociology*. Lagos, RMDS, 103–13.

Owumi, B. E. (1993). Traditional practitioners (healers and healing practices). In Oke, E.A. and Owumi, B.E. (eds). *Readings in Medical Sociology.* Lagos, RMDS Publisher, 68–76.

Weikang, Fu. (1985). *Traditional Chinese Medicine and Pharmacology*. Foreign Languages Press.

NOTES

Primary data collected from the following key informants. Are all anonymized.

Mrs. Adesina, R. O. (2009, May 15). She is a nurse who works in State Hospital Oyo.

Mrs. Nihinlola, E. T. (2009, May 15). She is a nurse who works in State Hospital Oyo.

Mrs. Oguntade, A. O. (2009, May 16). She is a nurse who works in State Hospital Oyo.

Mrs. Ogunyale, M. A. (2009, May 11). She resides in Elekaara, Ilora. She is a trado-herbal medics practitioner.

Mrs. Oyebisi, E. O. (2009, May 15). She is a nurse who works in State Hospital Oyo.

Mrs. Oyekan, T. A. (2009, May 15). She is a nurse who works in State Hospital Oyo.

Chapter 4

Health Care in Marginal Communities

Experiences of the Chronically Ill in Rural Zimbabwe

Alex Asakitikpi and Wendy Savieri

INTRODUCTION

Over the years, more resources and policies have been engaged by government and policymakers to fight communicable diseases such as malaria, the human immunodeficiency virus (HIV), and tuberculosis (TB), which are the leading causes of deaths in sub-Saharan Africa, leaving other diseases with poor attention. This skewed approach has led to the rise of noncommunicable diseases such as hypertension, arthritis, heart disease, cancer, and diabetes, as they are among the diseases that have received the poor attention of governments in favor of fighting bigger disease threats such as HIV (Boutayeb, 2014). According to the World Health Organization (WHO), noncommunicable chronic diseases will become the major killer in Africa in years to come (WHO, 2018). It is forecasted that by 2030, chronic diseases will account for 42 percent of all deaths in sub-Saharan Africa, rising from the current 25 percent (WHO, 2018). Although the rates of chronic diseases are high, as of 2009 only a few health-care systems can meet the requirements of people with chronic diseases, particularly poor patients whose resources to seek regular care are limited (Goudge et al., 2009, p. 1). People who live in rural areas are among the population group that experiences significant health-care problems primarily because rural areas are marginalized with regards to the provision of social amenities including health-care services. Rural residents are characterized by people who are poorer, are older, and have fewer health-care providers to care for them, and hence this is the reason health care is a major concern for people living in rural areas (Wang et al., 2014). This scenario remains unchanged till present.

Zimbabwe has been experiencing severe social and economic challenges due to international sanctions imposed on the country since 2002. As a result, the provision of social amenities has been neglected, leading to unprecedented deterioration of health-care infrastructure, the migration of experienced health sector personnel, and a decline in the quality of health services that are available to the population (Mangundu, Roets & Van Rensberg, 2020). In the face of rising chronic diseases, limited access to health care is a crucial factor to health care services among people living in rural Zimbabwe. Importantly, the adult population who suffers from chronic diseases such as arthritis, hypertension, tuberculosis, and diabetes face significant barriers in accessing health-care services (Nhapi, 2019). For people living with cancer and diabetes, linkage to care after diagnosis is a challenge within the cascade of continuum of care. The population that is largely affected by lack of access to health-care services is commonly the people who live in rural areas and have low income and a limited Western education (Tanser, 2006, p. 691). Even those who can afford medication must face the burden of travelling long distances to access health-care facilities and services (Arcury et al., 2005: 38; Mangundu, Roets, & Van Rensberg, 2020). The dwindling economic fortune of Zimbabwe also impacts budgetary allocation to rural communities, which also means that chronic diseases such as cancer, cardiovascular problems, and diabetes cannot be subsidized by the government. Therefore, most people who are suffering from chronic diseases in rural communities have limited access to health-care services and where available have difficulties gaining access due to the high costs associated with services and medication. Hence, decisions to seek care among people with chronic diseases in rural areas have been determined by opportunities to seek care, especially concerning time, distance, availability, and cost. This chapter reports on the lived experiences of chronically ill adults to understand how they cope with access to health services in the Mutoko rural area of Zimbabwe.

CHRONIC DISEASES AND ACCESS TO HEALTH-CARE SERVICES

Within the context of chronic diseases and access to health-care services, studies have consistently shown that people with chronic diseases often require frequent clinic visits, access to medication, and changes to treatment plans to provide evidence-based care (Hernandez et al., 2009; Longman et al., 2012;

Hudon et al., 2017, Chang et al., 2019; Verngust et al., 2017; Mangundu et al., 2020). For example, Hernandez et al. (2009) reported that chronic diseases such as cancer, cardiovascular diseases and obstructive pulmonary disease were associated with an average of 30 percent increase in health-care visitation and a hospitalization rate of over 50 percent yearly. Similarly, Hudon et al. (2017), in their study, found out that a significant number of their study population in Canada who were identified with chronic diseases were associated with an increased risk of chronic frequent emergency department utilization. More specifically to rural and marginalized communities, Mangundu et al. (2020) have reported that in rural Zimbabwe, the increase in the utilization of health services, including by the chronically ill, has contributed to the burden of the limited health personnel in marginalized areas of the country. Besides the increasing demands for health-care services in rural areas, transportation has been one of the barriers limiting access to health care, as most patients are not able to get their medication on time, while others are not able to get to their medical appointments on time, and some face the problem of delayed care (Cossman, James, and Wolf, 2017). The consequences of lack of transportation usually end up leading to poor management of chronic illness and hence poorer health outcomes. In Zimbabwe, the health-care system has been steadily declining, and as a result there has been a systematic decrease in the coverage of most basic services, and the mortality rate of chronic diseases has continued to rise (Chuma et al., 2007, p. 673). This decline has been evident in rural areas (Mangundu, Roets, & Van Rensberg, 2020). In the face of economic adversity, for many people, traditional and orthodox consultations now appear to be equally an effective health-seeking solution due to limited options. The determinants of patients' choice of medical provider in relation to poor access to health care in the time of increasing economic hardships have also been reported (Brundisini, 2013, p. 15).

DETERMINANTS OF HEALTH-SEEKING BEHAVIOUR IN RURAL AREAS

Researchers who are interested in the health-seeking behavior among the chronically ill in rural communities have identified several factors that are associated with accessing health facilities. Long distance to health centers, as a barrier, is a common deterrent to the utilization of health-care services by people with chronic diseases. In a qualitative study conducted in South Africa, respondents complained that there was no transportation to health-care facilities, and they had to walk ten to twenty-five kilometers before they could access health-care facilities (Pronyk et al., 2001). Similarly, there are no good roads in rural areas in Zimbabwe, which makes it difficult for the chronically ill and the aged to get around these areas and it often takes a long time before people get to health centers. Researchers have indicated that physical distance has a great influence on how patients perceive and experience health services and, in the process, seek health services (Ahmed et al., 2015). In a descriptive study that was conducted on how age influenced health-seeking behavior among chronic patients, with distance as one of its variables, it was indicated that some elderly men and women who are sixty years and above were too weak to walk to health facilities (Hong et al., 2006). Hence, due to old age, the elderly who suffer from chronic diseases do not have the physical strength to walk long distances to and from health facilities, and because of this, they end up staying at home and hope to get better rather than go to a health facility (Ayers and Kronenfeld, 2007). These findings demonstrate how distance alone can determine an individual's intention and motivation in seeking health-care services.

Reviews on the literature have also revealed that health-seeking and cost burdens depend on the type of illness. Chronic conditions such as HIV, tuberculosis, cancer, and diabetes impose significant financial constraints on households (van der Hoeven, Kruger, & Greef, 2012). Based on their reviews, van der Hoeven et al. (2012) highlight that health-services limitations, such as low reliability and coverage, user charges, and poor quality of care, contribute to high costs for chronic patients in rural areas, as the money they pay is not commensurate with the quality of services they receive. In Tanzania, for example, there are shortages of medical equipment in rural areas, and patients end up getting referred to urban centres for further check-ups; however, most people prefer to stay at home than seek health care due to the high cost. Van der Hoeven et al. (2012) contend that chronic diseases disproportionally affect the poor as they face difficulties in trying to access health care, and this has a great influence on their motivation and intention to seek health care. Studies conducted in Zimbabwe have also highlighted the high financial costs on the poor, and based on the economic levels in the country, the burden is not sustainable for many households, especially those residing in marginalized communities (Brundisini, 2013). However, this situation is not peculiar to African societies. A study conducted in Pakistan for example, found that the cost of seeking health care for people with chronic diseases with money from their own salaries meant using almost 85 percent of their families' source of livelihood (Shaikh & Hatcher, 2004). Such studies demonstrate that the higher the cost of health services, the less chronically ill people are likely to seek health care. There is also evidence in the Global North that shows that people who cannot pay for health services with other means besides out-of-pocket money may not be able to access health care when they need it (Brundisini, 2013; Hernandez et al., 2009).

In addition to accessibility and financial factors, cultural factors play a significant role in influencing health-seeking behavior among people with chronic diseases. In a study conducted in Uganda, it was found that in rural areas, there is little or no knowledge about diabetes and arthritis. Many people therefore attribute these chronic conditions to the influence of the supernatural, which means that people end up practicing limited self-care measures and do not seek professional help about their health; instead they seek spiritual guidance (Puchalski, et al., 2014). In a study conducted in South Africa, it was reported that spiritual care provides hope for patients with HIV because they perceive it to be a hopeless disease without a cure, and their belief that they need spiritual guidance motivates them to seek health-care services (Pronyk et al., 2001). In Zimbabwe, culture is an important aspect of people's lives, and it plays an important role in determining how people behave; therefore, it is essential to investigate how people's cultural beliefs in rural Zimbabwe motivates their health-seeking behavior.

Health-seeking behavior is a dynamic process whereby patients seek treatment from different health-care providers based on the type of illness and how patients perceive the severity of the symptoms of the illness (Cornally & McCarthy, 2011). Therefore, when chronically ill patients perceive their illnesses to be mild, they resort to self-treatment and buying over-the-counter medicines; it is only when the medication proves to be unsuccessful that they visit government hospitals or private health-care facilities (Delgado, Sorensen, &Van der Stuyft, 1994). The pathway model of health-seeking behavior is used as a theoretical framework for this study, and it is primarily an anthropological approach that uses qualitative methods of investigation (Mackian, 2003). According to Suchman (1965), the pathway model describes the steps of the process that patients take, from the moment they identify symptoms of an illness to the moment that they make use of health-care-providing facilities. This model will aim to examine and explain the logical sequence of steps taken by people with chronic illness in the Mutoko rural area. The steps are perception of the disease, evaluation of the symptoms, and the use of different care types. It also provides a framework for the analysis of how social and cultural factors affect this sequence within the context of chronic diseases, such as diabetes, arthritis, and tuberculosis, and how the social and cultural meanings attached to these diseases influence the decision-making of chronically ill patients to seek treatment (Mackian et al., 2004). This model is based on economics and elementary decision and decision theory, and the principle of cost-benefits is used to evaluate best courses of action (Fabrega, 1974). The principle of cost-benefits determines the course of action taken by patients. Since health-seeking behavior is a social process that involves individual interaction with the social network, it is important to look at the decision-making process of people with chronic diseases from the pathway model as developed by Suchman (1965). The model suggests that people's responses to symptoms are dependent on their cultural values or beliefs concerning health. That is, their perception of what is 'normal.'

Accordingly, the decision to seek professional medical help is either promoted or delayed by social factors. The improvement of the pathway model by Zola (1973) identifies five different types of incidents that trigger the decision to seek medical care, incidents that threaten people's notions of normality. However, the interesting feature of the model is that the decision to seek help does not necessarily lead directly on a path to the medical professional, as people may opt to patronize alternative sources, including traditional healers, religious homes, or other alternative home remedies. The results collected from the respondents highlight the processes that influence health-seeking behavior when ill and the choice of health service providers. Detailed analysis of the data, interpretation, and discussion of the results is given in line with the objectives of the study.

STUDY AREA AND RESEARCH METHODOLOGY

The Mutoko rural district is in Mashonaland East Province in northeastern Zimbabwe. It is a small town with a land area of 4,740 square kilometers and a total population of 12,500, even though it is only 143 kilometers from Harare, the nation's capital. Mutoko has a limited number of health-care facilities, and these include a few privately owned pharmacies, a private clinic, and a rural hospital. However, due to economic and political hardships in Zimbabwe, these health-care facilities have been significantly affected by the latter conditions, which has had an impact on the ability of the Zimbabwean government to provide public health care to most of the people (Chevo and Bhatasara, 2012). Mutoko has been severely affected by the HIV epidemic, and its prevalence rate in the region is approximately 21 percent, while the prevalence rates of chronic diseases, particularly TB, diabetes, and arthritis and heart disease, are 9 percent, 5 percent, and 2 percent respectively (Kevany et al., 2012, p. 51). Due to limited health providers in the region, people with chronic diseases lack access to health-care services. In addition to limited health providers, many factors like culture, personal beliefs, age, type of illness, access to services, and perceived quality of the services available have had an influence on the health-seeking behavior of the chronically ill.

For this study, seventeen participants were purposely selected based on their chronic health conditions. Once identified, the snowball technique was adopted to access other chronically ill patients who are forty years old or older. Interviews were conducted in the local Shona language after explaining the aim of the study to them and permission being granted by participants to conduct the interviews. Interviews were conducted in the homes of participants with permission for audio recording. After each interview, a transcription was made, and the narrative was subjected to a thematic analysis to understand the lived experience of the chronically ill in a rural community in Zimbabwe.

RESEARCH RESULTS

Access and Cost to Health-Care Facilities and Services

Physical access to health-care facilities was one of the most important factors that participants cited as influencing whether they sought health care or not. Participants stated that the health-care facilities were far from where they lived, and hence, they used home treatments instead of using health-care facilities. Distance and difficulties to find transport was mentioned as a primary reason why a chronic patient delayed seeking health care. One participant had to endure pain for two days, not because she could not afford the medical bills, but because she could not find transport to take her to the hospital. She indicated there was a long distance from their village to where they sought health care, and therefore, they had to use public transport to get to the health-care center.

> The roads in this village are bad, so there is a limited number of public transports that come to this area, at a scheduled time. This makes it difficult to find transport to get to the hospital when you need to get medical attention.[1]

Other participants indicated that because of the limited number of public transports, the use of private cars as taxi was expensive as they had high charges. Therefore, the decision to seek health care at public facilities was influenced by transportation costs, and participants had to use other means of health care that were available now, such as home treatments and the use of over-the-counter drugs.

Moreover, respondents indicated that because of the declining economy, they were not able to afford medication and prescribed drugs, which they perceived to be expensive, and this had a negative effect on their health. In the Mutoko rural area, people mainly depend on subsistence farming, and because of the declining economic situation, there has been a decline in the socioeconomic status; health care is not free, and everyone must pay for health-care services. The majority of the participants indicated that even if they wanted to visit health-care facilities, such as public hospitals, they could not afford to pay for the services because health care has become unaffordable. One participant who suffers from diabetes reported that sometimes she goes for a long period of time without medication because she cannot afford to buy drugs. In the discussions, the participants indicated that the reason for seeking health care was influenced by the affordability of health-care services. Another participant pointed out that if health-care services in hospitals and clinics were free, they would seek medical attention from public health facilities.

> If treatment at the hospital was free, I would love to go because I am sure the hospitals and clinics have the right medication that I need, but nothing is for free.

One of the male participants also stated that:

> At times, you go to the hospital, and they won't be able to help you, because of limited resources. This is difficult for me because I am diabetic and need regular medical attention.

Finally, a female participant noted that:

> The situation in Zimbabwe is now very serious, there is scarcity of medicine, and everything is now expensive, therefore, I decided to reduce my visits to the hospital.

The reports suggest that the major factors limiting accessibility to health-care facilities in this community is the poor state of roads and the absence of sufficient health-care centers to cater to the population. In addition to the distance to be covered to access a health center is the monetary cost of purchasing the prescribed drugs. Even though the majority of the participants favour public hospitals, the consumables are not free, and due to their poor economic state, their patronage of health services is compromised.

Decision-Making Dynamics

In relation to demographic factors, gender and marital status were given a considerate amount of focus by the participants. Most participants pointed out that gender influenced their health-seeking behavior, and men were the ultimate decision-makers regarding health matters. When women were ill and needed to visit the hospital, they had to consult their husbands first. As noted by one female participant, "I have to consult my husband before seeking for health, so he can give me money for treatment."

In the Mutoko rural area, men are the sole breadwinners, and they are culturally required to provide for the family. Thus, men had to be consulted by all members of the household to provide money for treatment. The men supported these claims and agreed that it was their responsibility to make the final decision on when to seek health care. However, some participants also stated that decision-making was dependent on the living arrangements of the families. As one male participant pointed out:

> It is me and my wife who make the decision. We both sit down and decide on when and where to seek for health care, depending on whether we can afford it or not.

However, this was different in the case of women who were widowed or separated, and from those who were economically engaged; women were more likely to seek health care than those who lived with their husbands, as they did not depend on men to provide or grant them permission to take decisions concerning their health. The decision process is therefore complex, depending on the final position of the household, especially of the man, the severity of the illness, and other factors such availability of health personnel and medications at the health center. Sometimes, decisions sometimes go beyond the immediate family. Regarding chronic diseases such as diabetes and hypertension, for example, participants reported they had to seek advice from other family members besides the immediate before seeking treatment. Participants pointed out that extended family members sometimes offered suggestions with regards to health-care costs and to some extent gave advice on where to seek alternative health care. As noted by one of the participants who suffers from diabetes:

> When I got ill, I didn't go to the hospital straightaway, as I needed advice from my husband and family first. My relatives and my husband refused for me to go to the hospital, they told me they would first use traditional herbs on me.

A few participants opted to seek health care based on the advice they received within the family and from the community. In this community, ignoring the advice given by the elders is frowned upon, especially by married women whose husbands have limited financial power to make independent decisions. Such women are usually at the mercy of the extended family, with little choice for them to make decisions that will benefit them. This means the decision to seek health care is not made by the individual alone, but by members of the extended family. Therefore, chronically ill patients may be forced to patronize traditional healers even if it is against their wish or they were less likely to receive proper treatment and needed to visit the hospital. As one the respondents quipped,

> Sometimes elderly people may advise you to visit the traditional healer or visit the hospital, and you always have to follow what they advise you even if you don't agree with it because if you don't, it will be considered being disrespectful.

Religious beliefs also play a role in the decision-making process, which in turn influence the health-seeking behavior of chronic patients. Some participants pointed out that they believe that "people do not just get ill" because they have contracted a virus or a bacterium; people get ill because of witchcraft. They reported this is the reason they get treatment from traditional healers—because they know they can give them the herbs that will keep evil spirits from attacking them. One participant who suffers from hypertension said that when she first experienced her symptoms, she thought she was being attacked by evil spirits, and therefore instead of going to the hospital, she visited a religious home for prayers.

> When I first experienced my symptoms, I was at home, sleeping and couldn't breathe and felt suffocated. I thought it was some form of witchcraft attack, so I had to visit a traditional healer for spiritual guidance. It was only when the symptoms persisted that I had to seek medical help from professionals.

Another participant commented that in their church, they are not allowed to visit the hospital, and therefore in times of ill health, they go to the high priest for prayers and to get cleansed of bad omens. Diabetes was one of the chronic conditions that was associated with bad omens and witchcraft. She highlighted that she used mainly prayers to improve her health.

Study participants also mentioned that stigmatization influenced their decision to seek health care. Most tuberculosis participants perceived that if people knew that they had TB, they would isolate them and think less of them; therefore, they felt embarrassed to seek health care. One elderly participant reported that he concealed the fact that he had TB and delayed seeking health care because he assumed he would not feel accepted by the society and his wife would not be willing to engage in sexual activities with him: "In my society, people mostly associate TB with HIV/AIDS, so I thought if they knew I was infected they would treat me differently."

For other participants, the main reason they were reluctant to seek health care was because they thought they were making a public statement about their illness. Participants expressing this view stated that TB was a shameful illness as it was considered by members of the community to be contracted by people who were unfaithful to their spouses.

Key Steps Taken by the Chronically Ill in Their Management

The severity of symptoms was one of the reasons chronically ill patients sought health care. Most participants reported that they had to evaluate the discomfort and severity of symptoms before seeking any form of help. A female participant indicated how perceived severity of symptoms determines whether to seek health care or not, which often led to a delay in seeking health care. She commented that:

> Before I was diagnosed with arthritis, every time I felt pain in my legs, I brushed it off and blamed it on the hard work that I do in the fields. It was only when my legs became swollen, and I couldn't walk that I decided to seek health care.

People seek health care when they realize that the pain has become too hard to bear or it affects their livelihood. Moreso, other participants reported that they did not realize the gravity of their symptoms, and therefore they delayed seeking treatment. One woman, a TB patient, stated that she stayed at home for more than four weeks without seeking treatment because she thought she would feel better in no time. She explained her experience in detail.

> When I started coughing, I thought it was a cold and it would go away, therefore I did not take it seriously. For four weeks, I noticed that the symptoms had started to progress and by this time I was coughing blood and the cough was very painful, that was when I decided I had to seek treatment.

Other participants agreed and suggested that symptoms such as coughing, fever, and chills were considered as normal problems caused by the weather or working too much, and therefore treatment was not necessary. Limited knowledge on the causes of chronic diseases and lack of recognition of symptoms implied that patients were more likely to delay seeking health care.

Participants reported that they must compare the level of the severity of illness with the cost of benefits; that is, they must balance the cost of benefits against the impact the symptoms will have on their quality of life. Participants indicated that their reason for seeking treatment based on the cost of benefits was both direct and indirect. One of the obvious costs mentioned by most of the participants was cost of care. They stated that the amount of money they had to spend on health providers would cost them almost a quarter of the family's monthly income. According to one of the male participants,

> For me to just book an appointment with a general practitioner at the clinic, I have to pay $10 consultation fee and almost $40 for the medication at the pharmacy and this leaves a strain on my family's monthly budget.

The study found that participants must wait for more severe symptoms before visiting health providers to save money. In addition, another indirect cost the participants discussed was the time they had to spend with health providers. Participants stated that sometimes they must wait in long queues for long hours at the clinic without being attended to. The long hours they spend at the health providers meant they were not able to work, and this affected their quality of life. For other participants, they must stay at home and work instead of seeking treatment as they do not have anyone to do the domestic and farm work for them.

> I am a widow with three children that I must take care of. I find it better to stay at home and try to provide for my family than to go and seek treatment as it disrupts my way of life.

Only a few participants who had family support and other people to take care of their families reported that they sought treatment as soon as they experienced any symptoms.

Patterns of Engaging Health-Care Services

The patterns of engaging health services among chronically ill patients were based on the cost of benefits, evaluation of symptoms, and the perceived preventive potential. When they perceived the symptoms as not serious, they engaged in self-treatment, and when that did not seem to work, and the illness remained persistent, that is when they used other alternatives, depending on how they perceived the illness.

Participants reported lacking information on regular checkups to monitor the onset of diseases or their progression. Instead, they monitored the illness at home, using self-medication that would come in form of painkillers, over-the-counter drugs, or other traditional concoctions to ease the pain. They highlighted that self-medication was for mild symptoms, such as headaches, tiredness, and fever. However, in cases where their health started to deteriorate or did not show any signs of improvement, that is when they had to use other alternatives, such as seeking treatment from hospitals or visiting traditional healers. One of the female participants in her fifties commented that "I monitor my condition at home, I look out for symptoms such as tiredness, headaches, and fever, and I use painkillers to relieve the pain."

A forty-five-year-old participant emphasized that when self-treatment fails the other alternative they considered was visiting religious homes. "When I used self-treatment and still failed to notice any improvement, that is when I sought prayers from a religious home that is nearby."

Some participants highlighted that they used prescriptions they received from the hospital previously. They did not find it convenient to regularly visit the hospital, when they could just buy drugs from the pharmacy using prescriptions from doctors and self-medicate at home. A fifty-four-year-old diabetic male participant stated this bluntly:

> Ever since I was diagnosed with diabetes, I do not frequently visit the hospital. I buy medication from the hospital with my prescription, and I monitor my sugar levels with a kit I received from donors.

For some of the participants, they highlighted that they visited health centers when they believed their illness was at an advanced stage, when the symptoms were severe, and when they thought they needed medical attention. This was because they believed that Western medicine is effective, and the clinic had the right medication for their illness, and this helped manage their condition. To buttress this point, a fifty-year-old male participant narrated his story thus:

> I am diabetic, and when I first noticed my symptoms, I used self-treatment, and I used traditional herbs to try and manage the diabetes. However, when the traditional herbs failed to manage the condition, I decided to seek medical treatment. They were able to assist me, and ever since then I have been able to manage my sugar levels.

Diabetic patients pointed out that they could not just go and buy over-the-counter drugs and therefore they had to visit a health specialist and get a prescription that best suited their diabetes type. Another participant commented that, "Some diseases, such as TB and diabetes, are difficult to manage without the assistance of professional health personnel, and therefore, using public hospitals is the best alternative."

Furthermore, as noted earlier in the study, participants pointed out that the decision to seek help from a traditional healer was motivated by the perception of the causes of illness. Other participants stated that even when they were in so much pain and in desperate need of medical attention, they had to think twice before visiting the clinic. A female participant in her fifties commented:

> Unlike the health providers at the clinic, who can walk up and down the whole day looking at you and without offering any form of assistance, traditional healers show that they care, and when they are not fully occupied, they treat you immediately.

Some of the participants stated that when they thought medical treatment was not as effective, their alternative was using traditional healers. They suggested that medical treatment and traditional medicine could be used interchangeably if the other was not as effective.

However, one of the male participants in his late fifties, who is diabetic, stated that he did not have faith in Western medicine, and therefore he preferred going to traditional healers rather than visiting health-care facilities. He commented:

> During the time of our ancestors, people did not use Western medicines and there were no hospitals, but they lived a healthy life. It is because of these Western medicines that many diseases are emerging.

Although some participants used traditional healers as an alternative treatment, others pointed out that they had never used traditional medicine when seeking health care. One participant pointed out that the use of traditional healers and traditional medicine was primitive and outdated. They indicated that they had never used any form of alternatives in their life when seeking health care. Participants who expressed this point thought it was irrelevant to use traditional healers in the modern world "where there are machines to diagnose diseases and a variety of medicine for any chronic condition." One of the male participants in his forties commented:

> Yes, traditional healing still exists, it is there, but it is ancient. It belongs to the older days, that is the reason why we now have hospitals. I am civilized and educated, and therefore the first decision that I take is to visit the hospital.

Other participants pointed out that the reason they did not seek health care from traditional healers was because they did not find their traditional medicine efficient. Their decision-making process was mainly influenced by observing members from the area who frequently visiting traditional healers, and yet their condition did not improve. "To be honest, traditional medicine doesn't seem to work on chronic diseases," says a woman in her sixties.

What seems to emerge from the result is that regardless of the obvious use of health centers for health care, many participants still reported that they explore alternative sources in their health-seeking behavior, such as visiting traditional healers and faith-based homes.

DISCUSSION

Long distances to and from health-care facilities are likely to increase the chances of patients deciding to opt for self-medication or visiting traditional healers, rather than visiting health-care facilities. In previous research, distance has been shown to influence the decision-making process on where to seek treatment. As reported by Bostock (2001), the distance to health-care facilities acted as a barrier to seeking health care. The negative impact distance has on health-seeking behavior is mainly associated with the cost of transportation and poor infrastructure. The infrastructure in Zimbabwe is bad, and the roads are damaged, and hence there is limited access to public transport in the Mutoko rural area. An increase in distance and a shortage of transport services implies some cost to travel to the health-care providers using private transport. Hence, physical access to health-care centers has a negative impact on the decision-making process of chronically ill patients as it is more likely to increase chances of not visiting health facilities.

The data generated from the study indicated that the socioeconomic status of chronically ill patients had a significant impact on their health-seeking behavior. The direct implication is that the cost of treatment at health facilities are high, and households in rural areas cannot afford the user fees and medication. This leads to a decrease in the likelihood of seeking health care. Agriculture has been left at a standstill in the country, and poor farmers in rural areas are struggling to get money for drugs. Hence, socioeconomic status plays an important role in influencing the health-seeking behavior of chronically ill patients.

The availability of health-care services also has an impact on the health-seeking behavior of chronically ill patients in rural Zimbabwe. There has been an increase in shortages of medical equipment and drugs in hospitals and clinics in Zimbabwe, mainly due to the economic crisis. Trained professional nurses and doctors are migrating to other countries in search of better job opportunities. Moreover, because of the sanctions imposed on Zimbabwe, access to drugs in country is restricted. This has left a strain on health-care facilities, especially in rural areas where people live with limited resources. The findings are supported by Chuma (2007), who found that there is an increasingly persistent shortage of drugs and lack of trained health providers in rural clinics in Zimbabwe, which has collapsed the health system. Lack of available health-care services in health-care facilities has left chronically ill patients without access to drugs and follow-ups from doctors, and this has had an impact on the management of their conditions, hence the reason they seek health care from other alternative health providers.

The study shows that gender is associated with health-seeking behavior of chronically ill patients; women must ask for permission from their husbands before going to seek health-care services. This is mainly because rural people have strong cultural beliefs in Zimbabwe. People have a common belief that a man is the head of the family and therefore has the final say in making decisions for the family. These findings are supported with a study by Lazarus (2001), who noted that men provide the main source of income and therefore are responsible for their family's finances and physical well-being. This indicates that gender has a significant influence on health-seeking behavior as women who lack resources to seek medical care depend more on their husbands to attend to their health needs.

Data also suggests a relationship between religious beliefs and health-seeking behavior among chronically ill patients. Many households tend to be more religious, and this has an influence on their decision to seek care from certain health-care providers. In rural Zimbabwe, people have strong cultural identities, and therefore when they perceive a disease to be caused by spiritual forces, they are more likely to seek traditional healing. However, religious beliefs may also affect the health-care decision-making process of chronically ill patients, because for patients from Christian backgrounds, they put faith in God and hope for a miracle, and in turn neglect to use medicines that will help them manage their condition. This concurs with other studies that have found that in rural areas, people have misconceptions about illnesses and their causes based on their religious and cultural beliefs, and in most cases, this has a great influence on how they respond to illness (Pronyk et al., 2001). This study found that some respondents' beliefs and perceptions of illness interfere with their health-seeking behavior, and this jeopardized their decision to access medication.

The source of advice on health care is also associated with health-seeking behavior. The majority of the respondents indicated that sometimes they must seek advice before any treatment. This is mainly because in rural Zimbabwe, elderly people are considered to have knowledge on certain diseases and how they are cured, and hence chronically ill patients value the advice given to them by family members and the elders in the community. However, because different people tend to have different opinions on where to seek treatment and on what works best in different situations, this is likely to leave chronically ill patients confused on what advice to take, and this leads to a negative impact on their decision-making process. This study found that this is because of a shortage of health-care providers with expert knowledge who can advise patients and give appropriate information on health-care decisions. This finding resonates with other studies that revealed people in rural areas often lack information on the causes of chronic illness and the appropriate actions to take, and therefore, they tend to turn to the wrong people for advice, and this has a negative outcome in the management of their chronic conditions.

Moreso, stigmatization is also associated with the health-seeking behavior of people with chronic conditions in rural Zimbabwe. Being stigmatized by people from the community because one is diagnosed with a chronic illness hinders people with chronic diseases from seeking health care. This is mostly common among people with TB, as TB is closely associated with HIV/AIDS. This is supported with a study by Scandalyn (2000), who found that society's beliefs influence how patients will seek health care. People with chronic diseases such as TB are more likely to delay seeking treatment because they fear being shunned by their families and members of the society, and this, in turn, interferes with their health-seeking behavior and how they manage their condition.

The severity of the symptoms and the perceived seriousness of the illness is associated with health-seeking behavior of chronically ill patients. Respondents who suffered from hypertension and diabetes are mostly associated with seeking health care than those who suffered from arthritis. This is mainly because people with diabetes and hypertension have a greater need for medical care. Respondents who did not experience severe symptoms were more associated with a delay in seeking health care. This concurs with other studies, which have found that the use of health-care services increases when patients perceived their health to be deteriorating. Moreso, people also have limited knowledge on how to recognize symptoms of chronic diseases. Chronic diseases progress slowly, and therefore having mild symptoms does not necessarily mean immediate attention is not needed. Therefore, hospitals should introduce education measures and teach people what it means to have a chronic disease.

There is also a relationship between health-seeking behavior and the cost of benefits. The cost of benefits is used to evaluate the best cost of action. Respondents are more likely to seek health care when the results are beneficial and do not interfere with their quality of life. However, when seeking health care has the chance of disturbing a patient's way of life, those who have responsibilities are more likely to stay at home and take care of their work and families, and seeking health care becomes second to their basic needs. This resonates with the health belief model, which states that individuals weigh whether seeking health care will bring positive or negative outcomes, and this influences their health-seeking behavior (Mackian et al., 2004). The findings from this study, therefore, suggest that the costs of benefits may hinder access to health care as people seek health care only when it is beneficial.

The pattern of engaging health-care services indicates that the way in which a chronically ill patient perceives an illness and the way in which they evaluate symptoms has an influence on the use of different care types. When chronically ill patients perceive the symptoms to be mild, they are more likely to use self-medication. When the symptoms of an illness are not severe, chronically ill patients tend to take a passive stance in managing their health conditions. This is similar to a study conducted in Tanzania, which found that households prefer to stay at home and self-medicate until they realize the severity of the illness. This is in contrast with some studies, which suggested that the main reason people used self-medication was because they could not afford the costs of health care from health-care facilities (Bennadi, 2013). This, however, shows that chronically ill patients delay seeking health care from the onset of symptoms resulting in deterioration of health until health care is sought from public clinics or from traditional healers. Thus, evaluation of symptoms has an influence on the different care types.

Furthermore, there is a relationship between the quality of health facilities and its influence on the different care types of chronically ill patients. Due to the economic instability in Zimbabwe, the quality of health-care services has been declining, and there are shortages of drugs and manpower. This was supported by a study by Mazilli and Davis (2009), who found that patients were not pleased with the quality of health-care services and therefore they sought help from traditional healers. This shows that patients are more likely to seek health care from health-care providers they see as convenient and effective.

In addition, the perception of the causes of the illness has an impact on health-seeking behavior. If chronically ill patients perceive their illness to be caused by spiritual and evil attacks, they are more likely to seek health care from traditional healers or from religious homes. Factors such as witchcraft, which are believed to cause illness and are beyond a person's control, have no link with biomedicine, and therefore seek people help from traditional healers. This concurs with a study in Uganda that found an individual's beliefs have an influence on how they perceive an illness, so if they perceive an illness to be caused by something in the spiritual world, instead of seeking professional help they seek spiritual guidance (Buregyeya et al., 2008). This has a negative impact on their health-seeking behavior as a misconception of the cause of an illness leads to a delay in seeking health care. This is because people have limited knowledge on the causes of chronic diseases, and therefore, they limit seeking treatment from professional health providers.

CONCLUSION

The aim of the study was to understand the lived experience and health-seeking behavior of chronically ill patients in a marginal rural Zimbabwean community. The study showed that the characteristic of rurality intersects with factors such as socioeconomic status, demographics, socio-cultural factors, and perceived causes of illness and evaluation of symptoms in the Mutoko rural area. Although participants highlighted the need for medical drugs for chronic diseases such as TB and diabetes, economic meltdown in Zimbabwe was identified as one of the major drawbacks in the management of chronic diseases, as hospitals have shortages of medical equipment, drugs, and health personnel. In addition, due to the poor economy in the country because of international sanctions, most rural areas are neglected by the government, including the maintenance of road for easy access to health-care centers, which significantly affects rural dwellers, especially those with chronic diseases. Policies aimed at improving the availability of health-care services and the acceptability by health-care providers as well as integrating traditional healers into the health sector may be a strategic decision to alleviate the challenges chronically ill patients face in rural Zimbabwe. This will, in turn, improve their health-seeking behavior as everyone will have an equal chance to seek treatment that they find convenient and affordable even in the most marginalized communities.

REFERENCES

Ahmed, S., Ware, P., Visca, R. et al. (2015). The prevention and management of chronic disease in primary care: recommendations from a knowledge translation meeting. *BMC Res Notes* 8, 571. DOI: https://doi.org/10.1186/s13104-015-1514-0.

Alazri, M.H. and Neal, R.D. (2003). The association between satisfaction with services provided in primary care and outcomes in Type 2 diabetes mellitus. *Diabetic Medicine*, 20(6): 486–90.

Arcury, T. A., Preisser, J. S., Gesler, W. M., Powers, J. M. (2005). Access to Transportation and Health Care Utilization in Rural Region. *Journal of Rural Health,* 21(1): 31–38.

Ayers, S. L, Kronenfeld, J.J. (2007). Chronic illness and health-seeking information on the Internet. *Health*, 11(3): 327–47.

Bennadi, D. (2013). Self-medication: A current challenge. *J Basic Clin Pharm,* 5(1): 19–23.

Bostock, L. (2001). Pathways of disadvantage? Walking as a mode of transport among low income mothers. *Health and Social Care in the Community*, 9(1): 11–18.

Boutayeb, A. (2006). The Double Burden of Communicable and Non-communicable Diseases in Developing Countries. *Transactions of the Royal Society of Tropical Medicine and Hygiene*, 100(3): 191–99.

Brundisini F., Giacomini M., DeJean D., Vanstone M., Winsor S., Smith A. (2013). Chronic disease patients' experiences with accessing health care in rural and remote areas: a systematic review and qualitative meta-synthesis. *Ont Health Technol Assess Ser.,* 13(15): 1–33.

Buregyeya, E., Kulane, A., Colebunders, R., Wajja, A., Kiguli, J., Mayanja, H., Musoke, P., Pariyo, G., and Mitchell, E.M.H. (2011). Tuberculosis knowledge, attitudes, and health-seeking behaviour in rural Uganda. *International Journal of Tuberculosis and Lung Disease*, 15(7): 938–42.

Champion, V.L. and Skinner, C.S. (2008). The Health Belief Model. Health Behaviour and Health Education; Theory, Research, and Practice. San Francisco: Jossey-Bass, 45–65.

Chang, A.Y., Gómez-Olivé, F.X., Payne, C. et al. (2019). Chronic Multimorbidity among Older Adults in Rural South Africa. *BMJ Global Health,*4(4), e001386. DOI:10.1136/bmjgh-2018-001386.

Chevo, T., Bhatasara, S. (2012). HIV and AIDS Programmes in Zimbabwe: Implications for the Health System. International Scholarly Research Notices. https://doi.org/10.5402/2012/609128.

Chuma, J., Gilson, L., and Molyneux, C. (2007). Treatment-seeking behaviour, cost burdens and coping strategies among rural and urban households in Coastal Kenya: an equity analysis. *Tropical Medicine & International Health*, 12(5): 673–86.

Cisse, A. (2006). *Analysis of health care utilization in Côte d'Ivoire*. Nairobi: African Economic Research Consortium (AERC).

Cornally, N., & McCarthy, G. (2011). Help-seeking behaviour: a concept analysis. *International Journal of Nursing Practice,* 17(3): 280–88.

Cossman, J., James, W., & Wolf, J.K. (2017). The differential effects of rural health care access on race-specific mortality. *Social Science & Medicine*, 3: 618–23.

Delgado E., Sorensen, S. C., Van der Stuyft, P. (1994). Health seeking behaviour and self-treatment for common childhood symptoms in rural Guatemala. *Ann Soc Belg. Med Trop.,* 74(2): 161–68.

Fabrega, H. (1974). *Disease and social behavior: An interdisciplinary perspective.* Cambridge: MIT Press.

Goudge, J., Gilson, L., Russell, S., Gumede, T., and Mills, A. (2009). Affordability, availability and acceptability barriers to health care for the chronically ill: longitudinal case studies from South Africa. *BMC health services research*, 9: 75.

Hausmann-Muela, S., Ribera, J.M. and Nyamongo, I. (2003). Health-seeking behaviour and the health system response. Disease Control Priorities Project working paper, No. 14.

Hernandez, C., Jansa, M., Vidal, M., Nuñez, M., Bertran, M.J., Garcia-Aymerich, J., Roca, J. (2009). The burden of chronic disorders on hospital admissions prompts the need for new modalities of care: A cross-sectional analysis in a tertiary hospital, *QJM: An International Journal of Medicine*, Volume 102, Issue 3, March 2009, 193–202, https://doi.org/10.1093/qjmed/hcn172.

Hong, Y., Li, X., Stanton, B., Lin, D., Fang, X., Rong, M., and Wang, J. (2006). Too costly to be ill: Health care access and health seeking behaviors among rural-to-urban migrants in China. *World health & population*, 8(2): 22–31.

Hudon, C., Courteau, J., Krieg, C., Vanasse, A. (2017). Factors associated with chronic frequent emergency department utilization in a population with diabetes living in metropolitan areas: a population-based retrospective cohort study. *BMC Health Serv Res,* 4;17(1): 525. https://doi.10.1186/s12913-017-2453-3.

Kevany, S., Murima, O., Singh, B., Hlubinka, D. (2012). Socio-Economic Status and Health Care Utilization in Rural Zimbabwe: Findings from Project Accept (HPTN 043). *Journal of Public Health in Africa,* 3(1): 46–51.

Lazarus, E.S. (2001). What do women want? Issues of choice, control, and class in pregnancy. *Tropical Medicine and International Health*, 2: 1175–79.

Longman, J.M., Rolfe, M., Passey, M.D. et al. (2012). Frequent hospital admission of older people with chronic disease: a cross-sectional survey with telephone follow-up and data linkage. *BMC Health Serv. Res* 12(373). https://doi.org/10.1186/1472-6963-12-373.

Mackian, S., Bedri, N., and Lovel, H. (2004). Up the garden path and over the edge: where might health-seeking behaviour take us? *Health policy and planning*, 19(3): 137–46.

Mangundu, M., Roets, L., van Rensberg, E.J. (2020). Accessibility of healthcare in rural Zimbabwe: the perspectives of nurses and healthcare users. *African Journal of Primary Health Care and Family Medicine*, 12(1): 1–7.

Mazilli, C. and Davis, A., (2009). *Health Seeking Behavior in Somalia-Literature Review*. New York: UNICEF & European Union. Report, 10.

Nhapi, T.G. (2019). Socio-economic barriers to universal health coverage in Zimbabwe: present issues and pathways toward progress. *Journal of Developing Societies*, 35(1): 153–74.

Pronyk, P., Makhubele, M., Hargreaves, J., Tollman, S., and Hausler, H. (2001). Assessing health seeking behaviour among tuberculosis patients in rural South Africa. *International Journal of Tuberculosis and Lung Disease,* 5(7): 619–27.

Prosser, T. (2007). Utilization of health and medical services: Factors influencing health care seeking behaviour and unmet health needs in rural areas of Kenya. A doctoral thesis, Cowen University.

Puchalski, C.M., Vitillo, R., Hull, S.K., Reller, N. (2014). Improving the spiritual dimension of whole person care: reaching national and international consensus. *J Palliat Med.,* 17(6): 642–56.

Samal, J. (2016). Health Seeking Behaviour among Tuberculosis Patients in India: Systematic Review. *Journal of Clinical and Diagnostic Research*: JCDR, 10(10): LE01–LE06.

Scandalyn, J. (2000). When AIDS became a chronic disease. *Western Journal of Medicine*, 172(2): 130–33.

Shaikh, B.T. and Hatcher, J., (2004). Health Seeking Behaviour and Health Service Utilization in Pakistan: Challenging the Policy Makers. *Journal of Public Health*, 27(1): 49–54.

Strecher, V.J. and Rosenstock, I.M. (1997). *The Health Belief Model: Cambridge Handbook of Psychology, Health, and Medicine*. Cambridge: Cambridge University Press.

Suchman, E.A. (1965). Stages in Health Seeking Behavior and Medical Care. *J Health Serv. Res Policy*, 6: 114–28.

Suominen-Taipale, A.L., Martelin, T., Koskinen, S., Holmen, J., and Johnsen, R. (2006). Gender differences in health care use among the elderly population in areas of Norway and Finland. A cross-sectional analysis based on the HUNT study and the FINRISK Senior Survey. *BMC Health Services Research,* 6(1): 110.

Van der Hoeven, M., Kruger, A., & Greeff, M. (2012). Differences in health care seeking behaviour between rural and urban communities in South Africa. *Int J Equity Health* 11, 3. https://doi.org/10.1186/1475-9276-11-31.

Vergunst, R., Swartz, L., Hem, K.G. et al. (2017). Access to health care for persons with disabilities in rural South Africa. *BMC Health Serv. Res* 17, 741 (2017). https://doi.org/10.1186/s12913-017-2674-5.

Wang, Q., Benner, S., and Leppert, G. (2014). *Health Seeking Behavior and the Related Cost of pocket expenditure for Chronic Non-communicable Diseases in Rural Malawi.* Heidelberg, Germany: Institute of Public Health, University of Heidelberg.

World Health Organization (2011). *The African Regional Health Report: The Health of the People*. WHO Regional office for Africa.

World Health Organization (2018). Non-Communicable diseases. Retrieved from http://www.who.int/topics/noncommunicable_diseases/en/. [Accessed on September 21, 2018].

Zola, I. K. (1973). Pathways to the doctor—from person to the doctor. *Social Science & Medicine,* 7(9): 677–89.

NOTE

1. An interview held with a male participant (X) in Mutoko village in 2018. He was fifty years of age. All subsequent quotations in this report were generated from field interviews conducted in Mutoko village in 2018.

Chapter 5

Family Planning Experiences and Reproductive Health Status of Multiparous Women in the Kisi Tsoro Internally Displaced Camp (IDC) in Oyo State, Nigeria

Paul Oluwasogo Omoniyi

INTRODUCTION

Maternal mortality remains significant for any nation, making it a major public health issue for many countries. Some countries outside Africa have experienced a decline in maternal mortality. However, in a developing country like Nigeria, a large percentage of women within reproductive age die as a result of complications in pregnancy. Thus, it is one of the countries contributing largely to maternal deaths globally. These deaths could be avoided if essential reproductive health services were available, including access to maternal and child health services that could help avert unwanted pregnancies (Nasir, 2022). Unfortunately, variations exist in the utilization and availability of family-planning services of which the contraceptive prevalence rate (CPR) is low (17 percent); thus, its coverage and utilization cut across northwest (6.2 percent), especially as it is applicable to women in internally displaced camps (IDPs) (Nasir, 2022). However, in 2019, only 842 million out of 1.11 billion women within reproductive age had access to modern contraceptives and family planning, while 270 million still have an unmet need (Kantorova, V., Wheldon, M.C., Ueffing P., and Dasgupta, A.N.Z., 2020). Unfortunately, this is worse for developing countries, where over 232 million women do not have access to family-planning services (UNDP, 2019). Nasir (2022) asserts that challenges exist for women within reproductive age engaging in family planning, which range from cultural, gender construction, and the power of men over women in the use of contraceptives. Moreover, women in internally displaced camps see the need for procreation as a means to ensure marital stability and as a form of self-empowerment.

In addition, cultural preferences exist for children and are seen as a means of competition for women when married to a man with so many wives, and finally, religion and poor communication among spouses counters decision-making by both parties. Similarly, Batista et al. (2018) is of the view that maternal mortality is influenced by the non-availability of health-care services in the community and the differing states of national health systems across the world. Family planning is described as the means through which women of reproductive age have access to information, methods, and means towards reproductive health services to enable them to control the number of children they may have. In sum, it is a conscious effort that allows individuals or groups to make decisions on desired children (NPC/ICF international, 2018; WHO, 2018a; UNFPA, 2019).

Contraception is referred to the use of artificial methods or other techniques that may help to prevent unwanted pregnancies before and during intercourse Casey (2018). Contraception and family planning involves a wide range of methods: condoms, pills, intrauterine devices, and surgical procedures, alongside other methods, which include withdrawal and total abstinence (UNFPA, 2019). Thus, the use of the above methods varies across young girls and reproductive-aged women as the former may utilize contraception for sexual satisfaction without been afraid of getting pregnant. For couples, it is used to control the number of children to determine the number of children to have and not be bothered with family planning. The influx of people into the IDP camps has caused overcrowding, paving the way for the spread of diseases, of which Nigeria is not left out with similar characteristics in its IDP camps across the states.

Amoo (2018) opined that overcrowding is the major problem, and thus this issue results in a situation where available resources are overstretched and are not enough, as well as the low availability of health services. Furthermore, the more people seek refuge in these camps, the more overcrowded and appalling it becomes, thus affecting women's psychological, physical, and mental health. Moreso, these persons are susceptible to ill health and other communicable diseases such as HIV/AIDS, cholera, malaria, and tuberculosis (ACSS, 2019; IDMC, 2018; and UN-Habitat, 2018).

The present insecurity in Nigeria has continuously increased the number of internally displaced persons, thereby putting many women and their children in a homeless situation. Presently, Nigeria, with over 3.2 million internally displaced people (Nnodim, 2022), is said to be the third largest in Africa

(Sasu, 2022). However, the northeastern part of the country has the highest profile in terms of internally displaced persons, owing to the war from jama' atul Ahlal-Sunnah lil da'awati wal jihad (JAS), who are known as the Boko Haram. Specifically, this region accounts for 2,171,652 IDPs as of March 2022 (IOM, 2022). As such, the rise among persons who are internally displaced have made internally displaced camps (IDP) a common thing within that geographical region and other regions within the country. These camps have been viewed as a means of succor for persons who are displaced, of which women and children constitute 80 percent of internally displaced persons (UNDP, 2021).

The crisis in the northeast and northwestern part of Nigeria caused by the Boko Haram terrorist groups have led to the displacement of over two million people (IOM, 2022). Women who are victims of violence, conflict, and natural disaster present in the IDPs have left their various residential homes and are left with no choice but to remain within the country's boundary (Emmanuel, 2022). Moreso, women are the major victims of conflicts and violence across the northeast (IOM, 2022). With the increase in IDPs, there is limited access to health services within the camp (Emmanuel, 2018).

Many internally displaced women have endured severe human-rights violations, which have implications on their reproductive health; displaced women are generally more vulnerable than other affected populations, owing to a variety of health issues (Mudasiru et al., 2019). Firstly, they are faced with psychological anguish as a result of being separated from their family and loved ones and are vulnerable to violence, including domestic abuse. They are also more susceptible to communicable diseases, like HIV and sexually transmitted diseases (STDs). As a result, women are also vulnerable to rape and forced prostitution, putting this category of women at risk of unwanted pregnancies, unsafe abortions, morbidity, and maternal fatalities, exposing them to dangerous situations (Olarewaju et al., 2019). Internally displaced women suffer from noncommunicable diseases, such as diabetes, hypertension, chronic kidney disease, and heart failure, as a result of poor health-service delivery within IDP camps (Mudasiru et al., 2019). These diseases lead to increased complications during pregnancy and risk of maternal death in pregnant women.

Similarly, poor health care in IDP camps has disrupted immunization/ family planning services, preventing women from receiving the human papillomavirus vaccine, which prevents cervical cancer (Paul, 2018). In addition, the lack of vaccine access increases the chance of pregnant women being exposed to measles and meningococcal meningitis, resulting in poor pregnancy outcomes. Without clean drinking water, proper sanitation, and great hygiene facilities, according to Burns et al. (2018), women have a tougher time living healthy, safe, and productive lives. Similarly, Mudasiru et al. (2019) opined that the rise of vector-borne diseases, such as malaria, diarrhea, hepatitis E, and yellow fever, in IDP camps is due to poor hygiene and sanitation caused by insufficient water availability. Pregnant women who contract these vector-borne infections experience miscarriages and other problems, which can lead to maternal mortality. However, these women have no particular provision for maternal and child health services in the camp (Olanrewaju et al., 2019).

More so, various IDP camps have now been established across various states within the country to help cater to more internally displaced people who seek refuge in southwest Nigeria, unlike in Borno State, where is it estimated that 1,613,019 IDPs are present (IOM, 2022). The resultant effect has brought about the shortage and unavailability of basic needs of life, such as food, water, clothing, and other medical supplies for women and their children across IDP camps (Emmanuel, 2022). Thus, women and their children are left with no choice than to be faced with several challenges ranging from extreme hunger, poor nutrition, disease outbreaks, high fertility, maternal and child mortality, and sexual harassment (Oyelude and Osuigwe, 2017).

In addition, insufficient numbers of health-care professionals and antenatal services exist for the diagnoses and treatment of possible pregnancy-related problems and other indicators relating to poor pregnancy outcomes. Maternal and child mortality is a result of inadequate delivery systems, PNC services, and restricted family-planning initiatives. Nigeria is one of the world's most conflict-prone countries, and as a result, internally displaced persons are forced to live in both official and non-official camps across the country, where they endure difficult circumstances in their quest for a better and more productive life. However, several humanitarian efforts have been channeled to IDPs in Nigeria, most especially in the northeast, and have received commendations despite the lack of funding. There is the need to bridge the gap in the context of IDPs and several challenges that are attributed to maternal and child health in the camp (IDMC, 2018; OCHA, 2019).

The aim of this study is to examine the family-planning experiences and reproductive health status of multiparous women in the Kisi Tsoro IDP camp, Oyo State, Nigeria, from the perspectives of multiparous women. This study is to help improve maternal and child health and enhance women's reproductive health status and needs through the availability of maternal and child health services in IDP camps.

The general objective of this study was to examine women's family-planning experiences and their reproductive health status in IDP camp. Underlying the above, this chapter discusses existing maternal and child health services available for multiparous women in the Kisi Tsoro Internally Displaced Camp. It also examines the unmet needs of the multiparous women's reproductive practices and examines the multiparous women reproductive health risks in the Kisi Tsoro Internally Displaced Camp. And the multiparous women's capacity to engage in family-planning decisions with their husbands in the Kisi Tsoro Internally Displaced Camp is discussed.

Thus, the need for this study is to document the experiences of multiparous women living in IDP camps. However, empirical data is still not available to document these issues, including women's reproductive unmet needs in the camp. These women often find themselves seeking shelter from one rural community to another in a bid to escape poverty, insecurity, and other forms of threats that are often more dangerous (Ishaku, Adeniran, Onyekwena, and Castradori, 2020).

CONCEPT OF MARGINALIZATION AND IDP CAMPS

Poor living and environmental conditions, coupled with the location and social exclusion of women in IDPs, have placed them in a situation where they lack adequate health-care services to include family-planning services that can help enhance maternal and child health. As such, women in IDP camps experience multiple problems in accessing health-care services. These women lack access to health facilities, and so many health care professionals have been put away due to insecurity, thus compounding the health crisis in the camp (Sambo, 2017). Lack of access to health and reproductive needs has led to the loss of IDPs from both minor and major health issues. Moreover, assessment from the thirty-six Displacement Tracking Matrix (DTM) asserted that 79 percent of IDPs are found in informal settlements that lack proper camp management, and they have uncompleted shelter, schools, slums, and no health services. These conditions put women at risk and expose them to harsh weather conditions; it also makes them prey for bandits (IOM, 2021). In addition, these assessments also showed an unmet need for water, sanitation, and hygiene (WASH) (IOM, 2021).

In the view of S.O. Adejoh, K. Irina, and D. Surindar (2022), marginal communities such as IDPs are faced with poor environmental health conditions and lack of access to health-care services, making people vulnerable to diseases. The accommodations provided for persons who are internally displaced often lack proper sanitation, including water and toilet facilities. About 40 percent of IDPs worldwide are found in Africa, a situation in which nearly seventeen million people have had to leave their place of abode at the end of 2018 due to wars, violence, and climate change. (IDMC, 2019a). In Nigeria, women in IDP camps lack necessary food, basic health care, and shelter (IDMC, 2019b). In addition, poor living conditions in the IDPs impact women's ability to procure safe food and avoid complications, infections, and other injury. Practicing proper hygiene, providing proper ventilation, and avoiding certain diseases is often not possible. (WHO, 2019). Thus, the issue of accessibility to health-care services for IDPs in this respect is similar to other groups who may experience poverty, as is evident in northeastern Nigeria, where 17 percent of the entire population, as compared with 23 percent of IDPs, lives in poverty (Admasu et al., 2021). Oftentimes, persons living in IDP camps known as informal settlements are neglected and don't have basic services delivered to them (Olajide, 2020).

Similarly, reports from the Brookings Institute in 2018 using the World Poverty Clock concluded that Nigeria is the world capital of poverty, with about eighty-seven million Nigerians living below 1.90 USD. This is evident through the standard of living of the majority of the people in the country, which is the result of the level of income across households and economic instability, which makes the case of women and child health worse, especially in IDP camps. Women in these camps barely have access to healthy nutrition, with just one class of food available to them, thus women's basic nutritional supplements are cut off, which are necessary for the growth and development of mother and child. Due to high levels of hunger and poor nutrition, mortality has increased for children under five. In pursuant to the above, women, who constitute the majority of the population in the IDPs, are grossly affected. These devastating conditions have contributed negatively in terms of life expectancy, maternal and child mortality, and other diseases for women. Cameron et al. (2019) used data from the 2010 Indonesian Population Census to compare MMR between high- and low-performing provinces. The research demonstrated the need to increase the health workforce to help address issues regarding maternal death. Also, it was observed that lower MMR in high-performing areas was highly associated with the increased availability of health professionals in a particular region.

Additionally, Sageer et al. (2019) connected persistently with the increasing rate of maternal mortality in Nigeria and sub-Saharan Africa to inaccessibility and underutilization of maternal health-care services, as well as a lack of well-qualified health personnel. Sageer et al. (2019) concludes that more than half of women who are pregnant in Nigeria do not attend the four recommended prenatal care sessions, and roughly 60 percent of childbirths have occurred at home since 1990. Moreover, despite the importance of postnatal care in preventing maternal fatalities, only around 33 percent of Nigerian women had received it by 2003. Meh et al. (2019) analyzed disparities in maternal mortality rates and factors using data from the Nigerian Demographic and Health Surveys from 2008 and 2013 among southern and northern women of Nigeria using multiple logistic regression. Findings reveal that low media exposure and a weak education system in the north and increasing contraceptive use and income index in the south, were major determinants for higher maternal mortality in the north as compared to the south.

This study was exploratory and cross-sectional in nature. Thus, a qualitative method of data collection was employed. Non-probability sampling technique was adopted using purposive and snowball-sampling procedure. Sample size was limited to thirty (30) participants due to the nature of the study. Data was collected through observation and inquiry using in-depth semi-structured interviews from multiparous women (IDI), health-care professionals, and camp coordinators (KII). This study was conducted in the Kisi Tsoro IDP camp of Oyo State. The choice of the study site was informed largely due to the increase in birth rate among women, but there was no succor for IDPs in Kisi Tsoro as it concerns family planning and reproductive health status of women in the camp. Thousands of internally displaced persons from the Benue and Nassarawa states have taken refuge in Oyo State, where their numbers have increased due to childbirths. Apart from food and means of living, one of the IDPs' major challenges is family-planning interventions (Daily Trust, 2019). The study population for this study was comprised of multiparous women aged eighteen to forty-five years, camp coordinators, and health-care professionals. However, data from this study was generated through a complex set of interactions comprised of women, men, and health-care professionals. Also, a multiperspective approach on family planning was generated from the study population and the disaggregation of the study participants by sects during the data collection exercise. This provided a more comprehensive picture on whether their experiences on family planning and reproductive health status are informed by religious, cultural background, geographical location, personal experiences, or individual interpretation and personal choice. Also, ethics approval was obtained from the Ethical Review Committee, Oyo State Ministry of Health Secretariat Ibadan. Also, verbal consent was sought from the women after the researcher explained the procedure, the risks and benefits of the study, and other considerations, to include voluntariness, confidentiality, and privacy.

THEORETICAL UNDERPINNING

This study was conducted using the ecological systems theory by Urie Bronfenbrenner. The theory posits that as individuals come in contact with different environments during their lifespan, they may experience changes in behavior in varying degrees. However, the individual environment is divided according to five different levels, which include the micro systems consisting of the family, religion community, friends, neighborhood, where the mesosystem includes the government, laws, political and educational systems, and the exosystem, which explains how the individual is influenced indirectly with the micro system. The macro system emphasizes the ideologies surrounding individual cultures, norms, and traditions of other subcultures, while the chronosystem explains historical and time influences. According to this theory, a person's society, organization, and culture are layered spheres, similar to nesting dolls. One sphere's actions can influence another (Rainberger, 2014). This notion is essential for comprehending the consequences of numerous facets of one's environment, which in this case includes all factors that influence the family planning of multiparous women and their reproductive health status.

Thus, it is critical to understand how individuals function in an environment that has a direct impact on their behavior. The benefit of employing such a theory is that successful initiatives at this level are more likely to benefit a large number of people in terms of health promotion. The ability to communicate with people about the phenomenon of women being the weaker sex, their status, and the impact of various aspects of their lives, particularly their reproductive health, will be crucial in examining the phenomenon of multiparous women in IDP camps. Furthermore, the conditions in which women find themselves puts them at risk and avails them the opportunity to engage in certain behavior. The unhealthy and unfriendly environmental atmosphere of IDPs is alarming and are affected by all that is within the environment. This theory helps provide a multilevel socio-ecological analysis and better illustrates the complexities that surround individuals in the environment where they live. The theory hinges upon the situation of IDPs and what behavior may be found among persons who are internally displaced. Birth rate is on the increase among multiparous women in the camp, owing to their conditions over time with no changes; thus, they are bound in an intricate web where there is no way out.

RESULTS

Socio-Demographic Characteristics of the Respondents

From the study, the socio-demographic characteristics included age, income, number of children, ethnicity, religion, gender, and educational level. A greater proportion of women in the camp were between the ages of twenty to twenty-nine, the majority of these women had two children or more, and a larger proportion of women of childbearing age were multiparous and only a few had a formal education. Most of the participants were Christians and were from Benue State. The majority of the participants engaged in farming as their means of occupation. Most of the participants had less income, ranging from #4000 to #5000. Understanding the socio-demographic characteristics of these women is of great importance as it provides other underlying issues that speak volumes of the study. These characteristics—for instance, age, education level, economic status, multiparity, and the kind of job they do—could expose women to reproductive health risks, and they are not able to improve on their health status due to their socioeconomic status.

Maternal and Child Health Care Services Available for Multiparous Women in the Kisi Tsoro Internally Displaced Camp

The findings of O.H. Okojie, E.O. Ogboghodo, and E.A. Omoijuanfo (2022) show that Nigeria is a major contributor for issues such as obstetric problems, postpartum problems, neonatal deaths, and stillbirths at the global level, more than any other country of the world. As such, antenatal care services are very important in enhancing women's health. Therefore, when women go for antenatal care (ANC), it helps to improve the health outcomes of both mother and child, which serves as a tool for interventions and programmes. Findings of the study revealed that women who register and attend antenatal services are less likely to encounter complications during pregnancy, unlike those who do not register, along with foetal mortality for women who do not book themselves for antenatal appointments. Thus, antenatal care services are very important for women during pregnancy, and the provision of ANC services across IDPs would help avert poor pregnancy outcomes for both mother and child. During prenatal care, women who have access to well-trained professional birth attendants can receive accurate and true information, particularly when it comes to mother and child health. Women are urged to deliver at accredited health-care institutions and are given the option to assess any risks or danger signs that may be associated with pregnancy (E. Abebe et al., 2019; G.A Fekadu et al., 2018). Every woman of reproductive age needs preconception care as part of her overall health care. The implementation of this service will help the health-care system shift away from procedure-based acute care and turn towards counseling-based preventive care (Akinajo, Osanyin, and Okojie, 2019). Maternal and child health services are not available in the camps, including antenatal services, which is an essential aspect of maternal services for women during pregnancy, key for monitoring mother and child health before delivery. As such, when it is time for delivery, women experience so many challenges. One of the participants corroborated the above statement in the following manner:

> We don't have any services available for women and children. See, let me tell you we have a challenge here that when women are pregnant or are in labor, until we go to Kisi, which is a distance from here, and if labor comes at night, even going to Kisi is a problem for us. I remember a particular man whose wife was in labor at night, we had to transport the woman on a motorcycle. It was

> only God that saved us that night because at times we would experience attack from Fulani herdsmen because of the distance. (Female/IdI/Guma LGA/24/Christian)

Access to Contraceptives

The study shows there are no available contraceptives in the camp. Thus, complications continue to arise from subsequent pregnancies. For some women, they are not even aware of family planning. Contraception is seen as the only way to help women to keep from having unintended pregnancies. One of the participants has this to say:

> My wives and I are not aware of family planning. If any of my wives would not agree to giving birth to more children, they usually advise that I can go ahead to marry another wife. At times, I maintain myself, but you know at times, too, we just have to give birth to more children as men. (Camp Coordinator/Male/KII/50)

Unmet Needs of the Multiparous Women's Reproductive Practices

From the study, multiparous women lack access to reproductive health needs, which includes lack of information during pregnancy and no family planning. The goal for family planning as a whole has not been met. There are 214 million women in poor nations who want to avoid pregnancy are not utilizing contemporary contraception, indicating that there is still an unmet need for family planning (WHO, 2018). Nigeria failed to meet the MCPR's lofty objectives. Women's rates are currently at 14.2 percent (FP2020 and Track 20, 2019b). Despite the fact that Nigeria has failed to meet its MCPR targets, the Reproductive Health Policy of 2017 set a target of 42 percent MCPR by 2021. Although 36.3 percent of the need has been met, 27.3 percent of the demand still remains (FP2020 and Track20, 2019b). Also, from this study it was noted that women in IDP camps suffer from preconception care, which is necessary and important for women, as this provides women the opportunity to address other health threats that may influence delivery and the health of mothers. One of the participants had this to say:

> Our antenatal service is once in a week, and we usually give education on family planning, adequate diet, exclusive breastfeeding, and the importance of personal and environmental hygiene, immunization, and postnatal services. Those with the threat of abortion are usually admitted, and during antenatal we do a routine investigation to discover persons with sexually transmitted infection like HIV/AIDS and Hepatitis B, except they come here. We don't usually go there;

> for some they go to visit birth attendants in town and are mostly referred here with complications such as postpartum hemorrhage, intrauterine issues, retained placenta, obstructed labor, anemia, IUFD, and so on. For multigravida, like eight or ten children are faced with untimely maternal death, and that is why we encourage them to go for family planning. (Nurse/30/KII/General hospital/Kisi)

Multiparous Women's Reproductive Health Risk in Kisi Tsoro Internally Displaced Camp

Edgal et al. (2022) reported that quality care from health-care professionals should be considered by women in choosing a place of birth rather than engaging traditional birth attendants with no formal training. Exposure of women to reproductive health risks include unsafe abortions, place of delivery, nutrition, socioeconomic activities, environmental conditions, hygiene practices, unsafe drinking water, cultural practices, birth control methods, and the utilization of traditional birth attendants. Despite the fact that family planning could prevent one out of every five maternal deaths (Okigbo et al., 2018), a study conducted in predominantly Muslim communities in northwest Nigeria found that more than half of the respondents did not use contraceptives because they believed family planning contradicted their moral, cultural, and religious beliefs, with no explanation given as to how their beliefs prevent family planning use (Adefalu et al., 2018). Preparing for pregnancy can aid a mother's ability to have a healthy child. Planned births have a higher chance of being healthy than unplanned births (Center for Disease Control and Prevention, 2020). Pregnancy-related problems, such as severe bleeding, infections, and high blood pressure, could lead to preeclampsia and eclampsia, which is one of the primary causes of maternal fatalities in Nigeria, as it is in many other countries in sub-Saharan Africa; others include unsafe abortions (WHO, 2019a).

From this study, we learned that respondents mainly use local herbs and leaves during pregnancy to aid delivery and avoid complications during delivery, owing to the long distances they have to travel in seeking health services. Similarly, findings show that women in the camp are willing to seek help but are disadvantaged due to lack of finances in acquiring quality health care. Thus, as expressed by a health-care professional, some women experience complications and poor outcomes as a result of local herbs used by most of them before and during delivery. Some say they cannot afford modern health care. Her statement was affirmed in the following manner:

> For some they use certain traditional medicine even before they come to the hospital; they usually don't like us to carry out investigation on them, which will help us, so they run away from the expenses because they don't have the

> money. Some babies are faced with intrauterine growth restriction, some have low PCVs, and the highest is 25 percent, 24 percent, or 27 percent, which is not normal for the mother and the child. (Nurse/32/KII/General Hospital/Kisi)

Other socio-cultural factors that may pose a risk to women's reproductive health are also discussed, which include early marriage, religion, and the cultural background of women. The study shows that women desire to have more children at a younger age because they believe that children serve as social security, and they must oblige to satisfy their spouse anytime any day. Also from this study, it was revealed that some men in the camp do not support their women engaging in family planning due to the perceived risk it may have on their wives. One of the participants expressed thus:

> For some women, they are not able to give birth again, neither would they see their menstrual period, so the fear is always there each time she tells me about family planning. (Male/IDI/57/Kienna LGA/Christian)

Similarly, from the study, the KII from a health-care professional shows that among certain cultural group, men are found to marry girls who are a very young age, and the young wife begins to give birth at that age. This is evident in the camps where young girls between the age of twelve and fourteen years are already giving birth. Culture plays a role towards increasing the desire to have more children, so the men marry girls at a very young age. This has implications on their reproductive health and may alter the delivery process when it is time. These findings were supported by a health-care professional, as expressed in the following manner:

> We usually see it among the Fulani, even among the Yorubas here, like the case we had yesterday. She is twelve years of age and the other fourteen years of age; others include thirteen and fifteen years of age. At that age, the reproductive system is not mature yet. Even during delivery, they won't cooperate for the procedure. For some, they usually take traditional drugs, and it has implications on their health. For some, they prefer going to a chemist to buy drugs, because they are usually scared of the several tests that would be carried out on them. (Nurse/40/KII/General hospital/Kisi)

Religion has its own role in family-planning utilization. Certain denominations don't believe in the use of contraceptives. As such, women are not encouraged to engage in it even when the need arises.

> Like for Catholics, Seventh-day Adventists don't engage in family planning. As for the Fulani, they mostly prefer to use traditional methods, and most

women visit the Traditional Birth Attendants (TBAs). (Nurse/30/KII/General hospital/Kisi)

Also, women's perceptions on family planning are influenced by other women's experiences, and the negative experiences and side effects of engaging in family planning makes it difficult for other women to believe in contraceptives.

One of the participants expressed her view in the following manner:

> Some of them fear the side effects, including unnecessary bleeding; some usually say they find it difficult to menstruate; they may be obese. Some, because of the experiences of other women, are scared of doing family planning. Some religions do not support family planning, so they don't encourage their women to engage in such. They would rather prefer to compete with other women. Some believe it will be difficult to get pregnant when they want to. An At early age, most ladies are faced with Invitro-Virgina Fistulas (IVFs). The government should provide us with trained health-care workers so we can engage in more education for these women. Health facilities should be made available to them, but the roads are also a problem—a major challenge for us—and lastly, there is a shortage of manpower in the clinics. (KII/50/registered midwife/Kisi)

CHILD SPACING

Many women don't engage in child spacing because their husbands just "pounce on them" anytime they want to have sex, and the women have no choice but to give them consent. One of the participants had this to say:

> My husband does not support family planning, and I don't have any choice. In my culture, some people see it as something good, while for some, they see it as something bad. For me, I don't want to get myself involved in family planning. I hear from some other women that when they engage in it, they find it difficult to menstruate. The government should provide us with good water; the water we drink is not good for our health. (50/Christian/Guma LGA/7 children)

One of the participants reported that in the camp, there was nothing like child spacing. They just produced children year after year, and even if they experience miscarriage, they conceive again almost immediately. Her statement is contained in the following excerpts:

> We are only giving birth here, and there is no spacing for the child. You would see a woman who had a miscarriage or stillbirth, and before you know it, she has been impregnated again. Though I usually have it in mind, there is no way. (26/Female/IDI/Guma LGA/Benue State)

Another participant stated she believed women should be provided with an education to empower them in taking up family-planning services. Excerpts from her statement is below:

> I have four children and have never gone for antenatal services before. Where I come from, they don't support family planning, and I don't like to engage in it. Women should be provided with education and empowerment so we can take care of our children. (21/IDI/female/Guma LGA)

Pain can arise as a result of women who continuously give birth to children without gaps between each pregnancy. One of the participants reported a situation in which some women experienced pain all through the period of pregnancy. She explained:

> I have given birth to eight children, but I had to endure pain all through the period of my pregnancy. I would love to engage in family planning, but I am scared of discussing it with my husband. If there were health centers around here, I would have gone there on my own, but, at times, we are even bothered with what we are going to eat so that we and our children will not die. Our children most times are looking okay because of just one type of food they are exposed to, and our children not growing well. Without the go-ahead of my husband, I cannot do anything or make my own decisions regarding my reproductive health. (32/IDI/female/farmer/Guma LGA)

Similarly, despite the complications associated with an increased number of births, some of the participants said that they desire to have more children. However, some women's cases are very pathetic with unintended pregnancies arising from cases of rape by bandits in the camp. This was supported by a participant, as expressed in the following excerpts:

> I still want to give birth to more children. I am still young, and I don't want anything that would cause harm to my health. During pregnancy, women face lots of problems, including body weakness and pain all the time. Many women in the camp have died due to complications during delivery. For some, they are not even aware when the baby is dead inside. There is a case of a woman whose child died in her womb after she was raped by bandits. It was not until three days later, when we raised money and took her to the hospital, did we find out the baby was dead. Even up till now she still has other health problems, but the doctor said it will cost money for the tests and we don't have the money. This woman was raped by Fulani herdsmen, and since then she has been the only one fetching for herself and her children. (20/IDI/female/Christian/farmer/Guma LGA)

BIRTH CONTROL METHODS

From this study, we can see that participants use traditional methods of contraception in the form of local leaves to prevent conception, although participants were of the view that a lack of knowledge of birth control methods was influenced by culture and religion. This was affirmed by a participant who states:

> For contraceptives, most our women use our local leaves. The leaves are usually joined together and inserted into the vagina to prevent conception. Many women eat guinea corn and yams, and this affects their health a whole lot. There is an increase in stomach pain almost for all women, and if we have a doctor here, we ask him to help us address this issue among our women. For women who marry at an early age, like fifteen years old, they are faced with many health problems. Some of them are not able to give birth on their own, and in some cases, they may lose their life and the child may also die. (Male/IDI/36/Goma LGA/Christian)

PREGNANCY COMPLICATIONS

From the study, it was revealed that women often experience issues of a retained placenta after delivery because they don't have access to antenatal care services during pregnancy. For some women, complications may arise in which the placenta will come out with the baby, which could lead to the death of the mother. One of the participants expressed this in the following manner:

> Women face various pregnancy issues. For example, the last time my wife gave birth, her placenta came out immediately, and she almost died because there was no way for her to receive antenatal care services at the hospital. If we were exposed to family planning, our children would be able to receive a quality education and grow properly. (IDI/Male/55/Farmer/Kienna LGA)

Women and children frequently die when there is no way they can get hospital care. The people seek the help of the government to provide them with good health-care services to prevent their untimely death. One of the participants had this to say:

> I plead with the government because through them all things will be beautiful for us. Our children have been dying untimely deaths, and we plead with the government to help us. The same goes for our women, who also die untimely deaths when it is time for delivery. There is no good health care, there is no

> good hospital here, and we seek government intervention. (Male/IDI/42/Oju LGA/Farmer)

Similarly, from this study, we see that women face problems during childbirth, and frequently access to the only place they can get adequate care—a hospital or health-care clinic—is hampered by their location, and there is no means by which women can complain of what they are going through when complication arises. This data was substantiated by the following comments from one of the participants, who said that:

> Before our women give birth, it is always a problem. The only option is to transfer ourselves to Kisi. My appeal to the government is to help us with a clinic that will help our women. My wife and I discuss family-planning issues, but the only option is going to a hospital, which we don't have here. The last time I took her there, they gave her some drugs and an injection, which I supported. Our major foods are rice, yams, and guinea corn. In terms of diet, we are only conditioned to just one food, and our women really complain a whole lot. (Male/IDI/31/UJU LGA/Farmer)

Findings from this study also show that maternal nutrition in the camp exposes women to a series of complications that may arise before and during pregnancy. On the other hand, access to quality food would enhance their reproductive health status. One of the participants narrated her experience of not eating food rich in proteins. The study also revealed that women lack food rich in proteins, like beans, to complement their meals, so they are left with no choice but to feed themselves and their families with what is available to them.

> Both in the morning, afternoon, and night, we only take guinea corn and maize; there is no way to balance our diet. I married at the age of eleven years, which has made me go through a whole lot because of the age I began to give birth. It has really affected my reproductive health status. I feel pain all over my body, and if care is not taken, I may still have to give birth to more children. I have six children, and I delivered them all at home. There is no one to provide us with information regarding a healthy diet during pregnancy unless we go to the general hospital, but it is very far from here. We are very poor, and we need the help of the government with maternal and child services. I haven't engaged in family planning. (Female/IDI/UJU LGA/25/Christian)

MATERNAL NUTRITION

The major foods eaten by women during pregnancy include millet and guinea corn, which is not good for their health. This also affects the growth of their children, making them look obese. One of the participants expressed it this way:

> The food we eat here is not too normal, so we are even confused. Maybe it is the food or the water that we take that is not good. (Female/IDI/27/Guma/Christian)

With an inaccessibility to pregnancy information, women are faced with poor pregnancy outcomes. Distance is also a major barrier in gaining access to this information. One of the participants had this to say:

> Women don't have access to information regarding pregnancy unless they are rushed to town; my plea is for the government to provide our women with health centers and a vehicle to help convey them, especially in times of crisis, when they are faced with delivery complications. Most of the women experience miscarriages. It is only by God's grace that we are living. We only get what we eat from what our farm produces, and that is the only way we survive here. (Male/IDI/36/Benue State/Goma LGA)

Our women face several challenges in trying to give birth, and most of them complain of stomach pain all the time. In some cases, women have retained the placenta during delivery. Similarly, one of the participants expressed thus:

> Women frequently complain of stomach pain when they are pregnant, but we don't get transport that would help convey them to the hospital, so in some cases we lose them and the child because of the pain. Some women have retained the placenta during delivery because here they deliver in the house and no proper medical care is given. We are resigned to our fate. For me, I have almost three wives, and we only survive from our farm produce. I married each of them when they were eighteen, and immediately they started giving birth for me. (Male/IDI/45/Benue State/Goma LGA)

Maternal nutrition is a major challenge. Some women are affected when they eat guinea corn, which, in some cases, increases the pain of ulcers during pregnancy. One of the participants expressed thus:

> I find it difficult each time I want to deliver; I have six children now, of which I delivered four in the house and two in the hospital. During pregnancy, I complained of serious stomach pain and eye pain, and I found it painful to lift any object or even cook for myself. The kinds of food we eat here affects me a whole lot, most especially guinea corn. I have ulcers, and each time I eat guinea corn,

> it increases my pain during the pregnancy. Most times I discuss reproductive health issues with my husband because of the pains I am going through. I try to make him understand, although he agreed to it so that I don't lose my life. I have already had six children at my age, and I am scared of dying an untimely death. I would love to practice family planning, but the distance is a major barrier, but I really want to preserve my health and keep my life. (Female/22/IDI/GumaLGA/farmer)

The kind of job they do also affects women during pregnancy. Most of them are faced with varying health issues, like high blood pressure, which is not good for mother or baby. A participant expressed this in the following manner:

> Most women, when under stress, are faced with high blood pressure, and that is a sign of eclampsia or preeclampsia. (Nurse/KII/35/Health Centre/Kisi)

Women often give birth in the camp because there is no means by which they can be conveyed to the hospital. So, it is a normal thing to do when there is no alternative. One of the participants had this to say:

> Here, we give birth at home because we don't have health centers here even for our children. Even right now I want to take my wife to the hospital, and I have been waiting for a motorcycle to just pass by. Till now I have not seen one. We see the way the women are forced to give birth, but it's normal for us since there is no other alternative. Since I arrived here, I only eat guinea corn and maize, but rice, beans, and other food items are very difficult to get. We find it difficult to eat a balanced diet. As I speak to you now, I have not even had breakfast. (Male/IDI/23/Oju LGA/Farmer)

DISCUSSION

Previous findings from Ndu et al. (2022) reported that there is a need for male involvement in family planning and vasectomy services. In low-resource contexts, the number of women of reproductive age who rely on vasectomies as contraception in Africa is less than 1 percent. The study focused on the need to address sociocultural and health conditions that may impede the integration and acceptability of vasectomies for family planning in Nigeria. Findings revealed that men are aware of the idea of family planning, but they are reluctant, owing to various factors such as fear, religion, and cultural beliefs, which prevent them from allowing their wives to engage in family planning. However, the implications of the above would affect policies and programmes aimed at family planning. This domination has continued to increase, owing to women being the weaker sex and being subjected to the head of the house, who is seen as the main figure when it comes to deciding the number of children the woman will have. Women in the camp have no equality or say when it comes to family planning.

Similarly, Okigbo et al. (2018), in their study, concluded that certain factors expose women to reproductive health risks, in terms of wife-beating, household decision-making, couples' family-planning decisions, and family-planning self-efficacy. This study examines the relationship between gender-equitable beliefs and modern contraception use between 2010 and 2016. In most societies, socially established gender norms, decision-making power, and resource control differ for men and women, with men typically having more authority and impact on women's decisions to seek health care (Sahay, 2018). Also, Adedini et al. (2018) discovered that church leaders' support for favorable social norms was a key method for improving voluntary family planning in Nigeria. Nigeria has two sets of abortion laws: one for Muslim-dominated northern Nigeria, and another for Christian-dominated southern Nigeria. Abortion is only legal if it done to save the life of a woman (Centre for Reproductive Rights, n.d.).

These intricate webs of non-medical effects, collectively known as the social determinants of health, combine to produce health disparities between and within countries (WHO, 2020a). They are the social, economic, and physical conditions in which individuals are born, grow up, learn, work, worship, and age, as well as the larger collection of forces and institutions that shape daily life situations (WHO, 2020a). Family planning is seen as the right way to go, even if there are different perceptions concerning it depending on the individual. It helps to reduce expenses by limiting the number of children in the family. The above supports the findings from this study, which shows that men are a dominant force over their wives, who are reluctant when it comes to decisions regarding family planning. The majority of men in the camp do not see family planning as the right way to go; in fact, some women also do not see it as the right path to take. However, one of the participants expressed his views in the following excerpts:

> Family planning is the right thing to do, because when you give birth to more children, it is an even greater burden on you. (35/camp coordinator/Male/Christian/farmer, Kienna/LGA/Nassarawa State)

Another participant stated that most men do not support family planning. Even if you ask them about it, their attitude towards the woman will be different. Even if as a woman, you are aware of the idea of family planning, when your husband does not support it, there is nothing you can do. One woman expressed her view in the following manner:

> As for me, I am aware of family planning, but I don't discuss it with my husband because he does not support it. (Female/IDI/54/Christian/farmer/ Guehi east LGA)

EARLY MARRIAGE

However, another participant reported an increase in childbirth in the camp owing to the fact that in the camp, young girls as early as fifteen years of age are impregnated, and subsequently this phenomenon spreads across the camp. So how do you expect them to know about family planning? She has this to say:

> Here, some of the girls are impregnated as early as fifteen years old. Most of them here don't even know what family planning is. (Female/IdI/20/Guma LGA/Christian/Farmer)

CONCLUSION

Findings of this study clearly showed the importance of family planning on the reproductive health status of women. From the study, multiparous women of childbearing age frequently do not have access to maternal and child health services. They lack access to these basic services due to their geographical location and their occupation. The women often cannot afford the cost in price and in time spent away from home responsibilities to access the services. There is an urgent need to make family-planning more services available to women in the camps. However, these women lack the vital information regarding child spacing, pregnancy-related complications, and nutrition that could improve the health of both mother and child. Relevant stakeholders must ensure that health policies are directed towards the provision of maternal and child health services. Women's socioeconomic status and access to health-care professionals are key in improving women's reproductive health status and child health, so efforts should be made to provide basic reproductive health services. Also, these women need to be empowered and encouraged if family services are to be utilized. Similarly, women must understand the benefits and risks of having more children and the importance of family planning.

In essence, women are disadvantaged, most especially in IDP camps, and as such, they are deprived from accessing family-planning services and decision are made by their husbands without their consent.

However, in closing the voluntary gap, women need to be empowered—especially women in marginalized communities, like the IDPs, where they don't have access to maternal and child health services. This would help reduce maternal and child mortality, improve birth outcomes, and enhance maternal reproductive health status. Governmental, non-governmental organizations, and other relevant stakeholders should ensure that women reproductive health-care services are given more attention in the IDP.

REFERENCES

Adebayo Adepelumi, Paul (2018). Psychological Consequences of the Boko Haram Insurgency for Nigerian. *Walden University Scholar Works.* Available at: Https://scholarworks.waldenu.edu/dissertations (accessed July 1, 2018).

Adedini, S.A., Babalola, S., Ibeawuchi, C., Omotoso, O., Akiode, A., and Odeku, M. (2018). Role of Religious Leaders in Promoting Contraceptive Use in Nigeria: Evidence from the Nigerian Urban Reproductive Health Initiative. *Global Health: Science and Practice*, 6(3): 500–14. Available at: http://www.ghspjournal.org/content/6/3/500.

Adejoh, S. O., Kuznetsova, I., & Dhesi, S. (2022). Internally Displaced People in Lagos: Environmental Health Conditions and Access to Healthcare in the Context of COVID-19. *Critical Public Health*: 1–6.

Adekanmi, A. J., Roberts, A., Morhason-Bello, I. O., & Adeyinka, A. O. (2022). Utilization of Uterine and Umbilical Artery Doppler in the Second and Third Trimesters to Predict Adverse Pregnancy Outcomes: A Nigerian Experience. *Women's Health Reports*, 3(1): 256–66.

Africa Centre for Strategies Studies [ACSS]. (2019). Population Displacement in Africa: Top 10 Countries of Origin. Available at: https://africacenter.org/spotlight/population-displacement-africa/.

Amoo, O. S., Smith, S. I., Ujah, I. A. O., Oladele, D., David, N., Oyedeji, K. S., & Ajayi, A. (2018). Socio-Economic and Health Challenges of Internally Displaced Persons as a Result of 2012 Flooding in Nigeria. *Ceylon Journal of Science*, 47(3): 229–34.

Asratie, M. H., Kassie, B. A., & Belay, D. G. (2022). Prevalence of Contraceptive Non-use Due to Husbands/Partners Influence Among Married Women in Ethiopia: A Multilevel Analysis Using Demographic and Health Survey 2016 Data. *Frontiers in Reproductive Health*, 4: 87–97.

Bagambe, P. G., Umubyeyi, A., Nyirazinyoye, L., & Luginaah, I. (2022). Women's Experiences and Perceptions on the Impacts of Maternal Near Miss and Related Complications in Rwanda: A Qualitative Study. *African Journal of Reproductive Health*, 26(5).

Bankole, A., Adewole, I., Hussain, R., Awolude, O., Singh, S., Akinyemi, J. (2016). The Incidence of Abortion in Nigeria. *International Perspectives on Sexual and Reproductive Health,* 41(4): 170–81.

Bashir, N. (2022). Beyond the Health Care Setting: Exploring the Intersections of Gender, Culture and Religion and their Influence on Utilization of Family Planning Services in Northern Nigeria. *Doctoral dissertation, Lancaster University.*

Bello, A. M., & Danasabe, A. A. (2022). Exploring the Implications of Forced Displacement on Sustainable Development Goals in Nigeria: Evidence from the Lived Experience of Internally Displaced Persons in Maiduguri-Nigeria. *International Journal of Intellectual Discourse*, 5(1): 293–306.

Bilyaminu, S. M., & Abughul, P. O. (2022). Assessing Environment and Sexual Behaviour of Internally Displaced Persons in Benue State, Nigeria. *African Journal of Humanities and Contemporary Education Research*, 3(2): 146–56.

Burns, R., Wickramage, K., Musah, A., Siriwardhana, C., & Checchi, F. (2018). Health Status of Returning Refugees, Internally Displaced Persons, and the Host Community in a Post-Conflict District in Northern Sri Lanka: A Cross-Sectional Survey. *Conflict and health*, 12: 41. http://doi:10.1186/s13031-018-0176-7.

Cameron, L., Suarez, D. C., & Cornwell K. (2019). *Understanding the Determinants of Maternal Mortality: An Observational Study Using the Indonesian Population Census Plus One.* https://doi.org/10.1371/journal.pone.0217386.

Cavallaro, F., Benova, L., Macleod, D., Faye, A., Lync, C. (2017). Examining Trends in Family Planning among Harder-to-reach Women in Senegal 1992–2014. *Scientific Reports*, 410(6): 1–11.

Dunn-Georgiou, E. (2017). Congo: *Faith and Family Planning.* PAI. 8 January. Available at: https://pai.org/blog/congo-faith-family-planning/# (accessed December 17, 2019).

Abebe, E., Gedefaw, G., Haile, Z.T., and. Ice, G. (2019). Association between Antenatal Care Follow-Up and Institutional Delivery Service Utilization: Analysis of 2016 Ethiopia Demographic and Health Survey. *BMC Public Health*, 19: 2–7.

Egal, J. A., Essa, A., Yusuf, R., Osman, F., Ereg, D., Klingberg-Allvin, M., & Erlandsson, K. (2022). A Lack of Reproductive Agency in Facility-Based Births Makes Home Births a First Choice Regardless of Potential Risks and Medical Needs—A Qualitative Study among Multiparous Women in Somaliland. *Global Health Action*, *15*(1): 2054110.

Etikan, I., & Babatope, O. (2019). Health and Social Assessment of Internally Displaced People (IDP) in Nigeria. *Annals of Biostatistics & Biometric Applications*, *2*: 23–28.

Family Planning 2020 (FP2020). (2017a). FP2020. *The Way Ahead 2016–2017.* Available at: http://www.track20.org/download/pdf/FP2020%20Progress%20Report%2020162017.pdf.

Family Planning 2020 (FP2020). (2017b). *Family Planning 2020 Commitment.* Govt. of Nigeria. Available at: http://ec2-54-210-230-186.compute-1.amazonaws.com/wp-content/uploads/2017/08/Govt.-of-Nigeria-FP2020-Commitment-2017-Update-SO1.pdf.

Family Planning 2020 (FP2020). (2019b). Over 2 Million Women and Girls are Using Modern Methods of Contraception in the Democratic Republic of the Congo as New Family Planning as Is Signed into Law. *Press release. 11 November*. Available at: https://www.familyplanning2020.org/news/over-2-million-women-and-girls

-are-using-mode methods-contraception-democratic-republic-congo (accessed December 15, 2019).
Fekadu, G.A., Kassa, G.M., Berhe, A.K., Muche, A.A., and Katiso, N.A. (2018). "The Effect of Antenatal Care on Use of Institutional Delivery Service and Postnatal Care in Ethiopia: A Systematic Review and Meta-analysis," *BMC Health Services Research*, 18: 1–11.
IDMC. (2018). "Nigeria—Patterns." Retrieved from Internal Displacement Monitoring Centre (IDMC): http://www.internal-displacement.org/countries/Nigeria #79.
Internal Displacement Monitoring Centre (2018). The Ripple Effect: Economic Impacts of Internal Displacement. Available at: http://www.Internal-displacement .org/sites/default/files/inline-files/20180608-idmc-economic-impacts-intro_0.pdf.
International Organization for Migration (IOM) (2020)—Global Report on Displacement 2020. Retrieved from https://www.internal-displacement.org/global-report/grid2020/.
International Organization for Migration (IOM) (2021)—DMT 36 North-east Nigeria Report.
Ishaku, J., Adeniran, A., Onyekwena, C., and Castradori, M. (2020). Building the Resilience of Internally Displaced Persons in Nigeria. *Centre for the Study of the Economies of Africa.*
Izugbara, C. O., Wekesah, F. M., & Adedini, S. A. (2016). Maternal health in Nigeria: A situation update. *Nairobi: African Population and Health Research Center (APHRC)*; http://aphrc.org/wp-content/uploads /2016/05/ Maternal-Health-in-Nigeria_ Final_Report.pdf.
Kantorova, V., Wheldon, M.C., Ueffing, P., Dasgupta, A.N.Z. Estimating Progress towards Meeting Women's Contraceptive Needs in 185 Countries: *a Bayesian Hierarchical Modelling Study*. PLoS Med. (2020). 17:e1003026.doi: 10.1371/journal.pmed.1003026.
Letamo, G., Navaneetham, K. (2015). Levels, Trends and Reasons for Unmet Need for Family Planning among Married Women in Botswana: A Cross-Sectional Study. *BMJ Open*, 66(3): 1–11.
Lwin, K. Z., & Punpuing, S. (2022). Determinants of Institutional Maternity Services Utilization in Myanmar. *PloS one*, *17*(4): e0266185.
MacLachlan, E., Agali, B. I., Maytan-Joneydi, A., Chaibou, S., Garba, S. A., Halidou, I. C., & Nouhou, A. M. (2022). Qualitative Assessment of Providers' Experiences with a Segmentation Counseling Tool for Family Planning in Niger.
Mayhew, S., Colombini, M., Kimani, J., Tomlin, K., Warren, C., Mutemwa, R. (2017). Fertility Intentions and Contraceptive Practices among Clinic-users living with HIV in Kenya: A Mixed Methods Study. *BMC Public Health*, 17(626): 1–15.
Meh, C., Thind, A., &Ryan, B. (2019). Levels and Determinants of Maternal Mortality in Northern and Southern Nigeria. *BMC Pregnancy Childbirth* 19, 417. Https://doi.org/10.1186/s12884-019-2471-8.
Mudasiru, S. O., Oladipupo, O. B., & Fatai, A. S. (2019). Conflicts and Insurgency: Barriers to Global Quality Health Service for Internally Displaced Persons in the North Eastern Part of Nigeria. *African Journal of Political Science and International Relations,* 13(4): 40–52.

Ndu, M., Nouvet, E., Odezugo, G., Dorayi, A., Okekearu, I., & Wallace, L. J. (2022). Barriers to Vasectomy Acceptance and Uptake in Nigeria: A Review of the Literature. *African Journal of Reproductive Health*, 26(3): 37–45.

Okojie, O. H., Ogboghodo, E. O., & Omoijuanfo, E. A. (2022). Maternal and Neonatal Outcomes of Booked and Unbooked Pregnancies in Benin City, Southern Nigeria: A Comparative Study. *Journal of Community Medicine and Primary Health Care*, 34(2): 109–27.

Olanrewaju, F. O., Olanrewaju, A., Omotoso, F., Alabi, J. O., Amoo, E., Loromeke, E., & Ajayi, L. (2019). Insurgency and the Invisible Displaced Population in Nigeria: A Situational Analysis. *SAGE Open*. https://doi.org/10.1177/2158244019846207.

Sajedinejad. S., Majdzadeh, R., Vedadhir, A., Tabatabaei, M. G., Mohammad K. (2015). Maternal Mortality: A Cross-Sectional Study in Global Health. *Global Health,* 11(4): 1–13. https://doi.org/10.1186/s12992-015-0087-y.

Sedgh, G., Ashford, L., and Hussain, R. (2016). Unmet Need for Contraception in Developing Countries: Examining Women's Reasons for Not Using a Method. *Guttmacher Institute.* Available at: https://www.guttmacher.org/sites/default/files /report_pdf/unmet-need-for-contraception-in-developing-countries-report.pdf (accessed on December 12, 2016).

Solanke, B. L., Adetutu, O. M., Sunmola, K. A., Opadere, A. A., Adeyemi, N. K., & Soladoye, D. (2022). Multi-Level Predictors of Sexual Autonomy among Married Women in Nigeria. *BMC Women's Health*, 22(1): 1–12.

Starbird, E., Norton, M., Marcus, R. (2016). Investing in Family Planning: Key to Achieving the Sustainable Development Goals. *Global Health: Science and Practice*, 4(2): 191–210.

Terefe, G., Abebe, F., & Teka, B. (2022). Unmet Need for Family Planning Service and Associated Factors among Homeless Women of Reproductive Age Group in Jimma Zone Administrative Towns, Ethiopia. *Open Access Journal of Contraception*, 13, 83.

UNDP. Costing the Three Transformative Results (2019). Available at: https://www .unfpa.org/sites/default/files/pub-pdf/Transformative_results_journal_23-online .pdf (accessed August 17, 2020).

UN-Habitat. (2018). The Right to Adequate Housing. Fact Sheet No. 21/Rev.1. Available at: https://www.ohchr.org/Documents/ Publications/FS21_rev_1_Housing_en.pdf (accessed December 29, 2018).

United Nations Population Fund (UNFPA). (2017). Regional Interventions Action Plan. .

Wekere, F. C. C., Enyindah, C. E., & Udofia, E. A. (2022). Permanent Method of Postpartum Contraception (Bilateral tubal ligation): Experience at the Rivers State University Teaching Hospital. *Age*, 25(29): 7.

Chapter 6

Reflections on the Sexual and Reproductive Health Context of Migrant Population in South Africa

Caroline Ndebia and Emeka E. Obioha

INTRODUCTION

In the year 2022, South Africa still remains one of the nations most severely affected by HIV/AIDS. In South Africa, there were an estimated 5.6 million persons living with HIV and AIDS in 2009 (UNAIDS, 2009). Younger adults were more impacted than older adults, with the prevalence rate among those aged fifteen to forty-nine years being 17.8 percent. Migration has been cited in earlier research as one of the main causes of HIV and AIDS, particularly in poorer countries (Lurie et al., 2003). It has been noted that migrants use condoms less than South African residents (Pfarrwaller & Suris, 2012). South Africa has welcomed a sizeable immigrant population from all over the continent and other continents over the years. In addition, the employment of migrant labor in South Africa dates back to the apartheid era. Previously, the rising rates of sexually transmitted infections (including HIV) signaled a rise in unsafe sex practices among migrants (UNAIDS, 2005). Females appear to have been the main victims of HIV infections. For instance, globally, the gender distribution of HIV infection among migrants shows that 59 percent are female, while only 41 percent are male (UNAIDS, 2007). However, with the prevalence of sexually transmitted diseases like HIV growing, the HIV epidemic has not significantly declined at a national level, but many migrants still believe they are at a low risk of contracting the HIV infection (UNAIDS, 2005). The high rates of risky behaviors, multiple sex partners, and less-frequent condom use, reported in earlier research, are likely to increase the potential for more HIV infections among migrants in South Africa (Kelly et al., 2003).

Two fundamental ideas—migration and health—serve as the foundation of this chapter. One of the key forces influencing the growth of the world economy is migration. However, this method has shown to be difficult and to have its difficulties, including negative health effects. This has damaged migration's reputation because it is now seen as an important factor in the spreading of contagious diseases, particularly HIV and AIDS (Brummer, 2002). Studies from around the world have found that migrant and mobile communities had higher rates of HIV infection than general populations (Bletzer, 1995). Thus, migration seems to be a significant factor in the global spread of the AIDS epidemic. Due to a variety of other factors, including being apart from partners and families, peer pressure, alcohol usage, low perceived HIV infection risk, restricted access to health care, and low levels of education, migrants may be more susceptible to infection. Younger male migrants from China who began having sex earlier had more premarital partners, more frequent sexual experiences, and more intimate relationships (He et al., 2005). Similar reasons prompted Nepali migrants in India to engage in high-risk sexual activities. These included meeting or exceeding peer expectations and pressure, cheap sex, a lack of parental control, alcohol usage, and a poor perception of HIV and other STD vulnerabilities (Smith-Estelle & Gruskin, 2003). Some of the major groups of migrant workers in Southern Africa were miners, truck drivers, seasonal farm workers, service members, and construction workers. They frequently spent extended periods away from home due to the nature of their professions, following a pattern of circular mobility between their long-term spouses and their locations of employment. Truck drivers and construction workers have also regularly moved from one site to another as part of their jobs in addition to this circular migration. Typically, migrant workers are placed in rural settings where they interact with economically marginalized women, some of whom engage in sexual encounters with them in exchange for material support for their families (Lurie et al., 2003).

Having presented pertinent background issues, this chapter proceeds with articulation on various theoretical reflections regarding sexual and reproductive health behavior, contextualizing migrants' vulnerability and risky sexual behavior, migration and HIV/AIDS nexus, perception of HIV risk, level of precaution and behavior change, and socioeconomic predictors of immigrants' sexual and reproductive health product use.

THEORETICAL REFLECTIONS ON REPRODUCTIVE AND SEXUAL BEHAVIOR

Theory of Planned Behavior

To predict and explain behavior that is not totally under a person's control, the theory of planned behavior was developed as an extension of the idea of reasoned action (Ajzen, 1991). Women's decisions to use condoms may be influenced by their sexual partners' participation and the power dynamics in their relationships (Bogart et al., 2000). The concept of planned behavior holds that the activity is caused by behavioral intention, which is impacted by attitudes toward a particular behavior, subjective norms (felt social pressure to carry out the behavior), and perceived behavioral control. The latter is concerned with both internal and external elements that may help or impede a person's behavioral performance (Godin et al., 2016), and it is said to predict intention and behavior (Ajzen, 1991). Underlying beliefs have an impact on behavior control perception, subjective norm, and attitude. People's ideas and assessments of the consequences of a behavior, for instance, influence how they feel about that behavior. The extent to which an individual feels in control of behavior (perceived behavioral control) and the degree to which that behavior is facilitated by the skills and resources one believes one needs to perform the behavior, together determine the influence of others on an individual's behavior (subjective norm). In other words, if a woman feels in control of her condom use, senses social pressure to use condoms, and has a good attitude toward using condoms, she will be more inclined to try using a condom (Ajzen, 1991).

Health Belief Model

The "health belief model" seeks to explain and predict health-related behavior by using specific cognitive patterns (Ajzen, 1991). The health belief model addresses people's perceptions of the threat posed by a health problem (susceptibility and severity), the benefits of avoiding the threat, and the factors influencing their decision to act (barriers, cues to action, and self-efficacy) (Godin et al., 1996). For people to take action, the Health Belief Model emphasizes that fear and self-efficacy must be balanced. According to Godin et al. (1996), the factors that led a person to alter their behavior in response to perceived threats were perceived vulnerability, perceived seriousness or severity, perceived threat, perceived advantages, and considered barriers (self-efficacy and cues to action). People must value and see their current behavioral patterns as a danger for behavior change to be successful. According to the perceived susceptibility model, an individual's impression of their susceptibility to diseases, their potential severity, and the availability of an effective strategy for preventing disease all have a role in how ready they are to take action for their health. The individual must think his or her health is at risk. The individual must think they can have an asymptomatic illness like HIV and not have any symptoms. Regarding perceived seriousness or severity, the individual must consider how significant the ailment may be in terms of pain or discomfort, time away from work, and financial hardships. Concerning perceived benefits, the individual must think that the change of a particular kind would provide the desired end at a reasonable cost. After evaluating the situation, the person must be persuaded that the benefits of the suggested behavior outweigh the inconvenience and cost and that they are feasible and within reach. We also have self-efficacy and cues to action in perceived barriers. Self-efficacy is the capacity to engage in the behavior required to effect results. The individual must believe in his or her ability to overcome real or imagined obstacles to taking action. Cues to action concern the relationships between occurrences, what causes what, and how behavior may affect results.

CONTEXTUALIZING MIGRANTS' VULNERABILITY AND RISKY SEXUAL BEHAVIOR

Literature from around the world has demonstrated that migrants frequently experience unfavorable socioeconomic circumstances that have a negative impact on their sexual behavior. It is commonly known that immigration status is related to risky sexual behavior. This observation applies to both developed and developing nations (Brummer, 2002). Studies on the relationships between migration and condom use as a proximal practice in HIV prevention seem to fall into one of two camps. The idea that migration encourages risky sexual conduct is one of them (Salabbaria-Pena et al., 2003). Breaking away from conventional care and supervision is frequently caused by being away from home and family. Yang (2004) asserts that those who have many sexual partners may engage in socially abnormal behaviors, like promiscuity and risky sex. This school of thought contends that immigrants generally take risks and are more prone to engage in high-risk sexual behavior.

The opposing school of thought contends that because of their migration, migrants are forced into unsafe environments where using condoms is challenging (IOM, 2008). According to research done in Zambia at the Chiawa Farm, women are occasionally lured or forced into having sex in exchange for employment, desirable jobs, or additional pay. In these precarious situations, it seems like condoms are rarely used (Bond & Dover, 1997). Men were forced to migrate thousands of kilometers away from their partners and families to work in the mines in the South African mining environment due to socioeconomic factors such as rural poverty and unemployment. Because these men were staying in cramped single-sex hostels and were frequently separated from their partners, many miners were drawn to look for a female companion who was easily accessible, close to the hostels. Miners were less likely to think about the possibility of AIDS, which would only have a later effect, but because of the hazardous working conditions, disease, death, and injury were constant threats for some for five to ten years (Campbell, 2000). UNAIDS (2008) contributes significantly to our understanding of the relationship between risky sexual behaviors and informal settlement. According to UNAIDS (2005), the host community, stressed migration patterns, and the host community's hostility against migrants, in which migrants lacked assistance from host communities, may compel migrants to participate in risky casual sex or sex employment. And in such risky casual sex, they are susceptible to HIV. This illustrates that immigrants' sexual behavior is affected by their isolation from the host communities; therefore, immigrants' integration and access to resources can help them avoid harmful sexual behaviors.

EMPIRICAL EVIDENCE ON MIGRATION AND HIV/AIDS NEXUS

Migration is correlated with both high-risk sexual behavior and HIV infection. Results have indicated that migrants report more sexual risky behaviors and promiscuity than non-migrants, which could have led to the high HIV incidence rates (Lurie & Williams, 2003). Numerous studies have attempted to examine the relationship between HIV and migration (IOM, 2005). Williamson (2004) specifically suggests a connection between migration and the risk of contracting HIV. According to studies on the connection between various migratory populations and disease in the Southern African region, migrants are one of the groups most vulnerable to HIV (Rijks, 2006). In a study of 196 migrant men and 64 non-migrant men in South Africa, Lurie et al. (2003) found that, respectively, 25.9 percent of the migrant men and 12.7 percent of the non-migrant men were infected with HIV. It was discovered that there is a sizable risk of HIV infection among migrants. Similar findings were made by Lurie (in IOM, 2005), who found that migrant spouses were more than twice as likely to have one spouse who was HIV positive than non-migrant couples. According to research, there is a considerable link between social support and safe sex (Campbell, 2003). According to Campbell (2003), when people feel lonely and alone, having a physical relationship with another person may come to represent an emotional intimacy that they do not experience in other areas of their lives. This is especially important for immigrants.

People often migrate in search of better socioeconomic conditions as a result of disequilibrium between rural and urban areas. As a result, migration has led to many problems such as overpopulation and crowding in cities, lack of employment, inadequate infrastructure, increased crime rates, prostitution, and other public health problems. Urbanization in sub-Saharan Africa, between 1960 and 1980, caused by rural migration, was responsible for the spread of HIV-1 to large population centres. In West African countries, migration was also responsible for the spread of endemic HIV-2 (UNAIDS, 2008). According to UNAIDS (2008), about 67 percent of the total people living with HIV/AIDS are residents of sub-Saharan Africa. Males tend to be more mobile than women, and they typically migrate farther away and for a longer period of time. This fact increases the probability of male migrants seeking other sexual partners, therefore increasing their risk of contracting the HIV infection. An investigation among South African educators also revealed a connection between mobility and HIV infection. When compared to educators who stayed in the same locations after finishing their studies (18.9 percent; 95 percent CI: 17.3–20.6), it was shown that those who migrated without their families to their place of employment after finishing their studies had a higher HIV prevalence (23.5 percent; 95 percent CI: 21.4–25.8) (Lurie et al., 1997). According to Zuma et al. (2003), immigrant women are noticeably more likely than non-immigrant women to have two or more lifetime relationships. As a result, migrant women are now at a higher risk of contracting HIV (46.0 percent, $p=0.011$) than non-migrant women (34.7 percent, $p=0.011$). Education is not a predictor of HIV infection, claims Zuma et al. (2003). On the other side, Zuma (2003) discovers that South Africa has a high rate of circular mobility between rural and urban areas, which is known to raise the risk of HIV infection in women whose partners are migrants. Thus, it suggests that migration is linked to the expansion and high incidence of HIV in Africa. Numerous research has looked into the connection between migration and the spread of HIV in Africa and other places (Voeten et al., 2010).

Although the majority of studies concentrate on international migration (Tranos et al., 2015), they are nevertheless pertinent to this study since, for the most part, both internal and international migrants encounter the same challenges when they arrive at their final destinations. Migration and mobile people in general, according to Brummer (2002), "have played a substantial influence in the initial dissemination of HIV in the Southern African region." In the same line, Decosas et al. (1995) asserts that while the presence of migrants in host communities has been connected to the spread of HIV, no instances of a substantial pandemic being sparked by the entry of migrants from other countries have been seen in Africa. He goes on to say that "the social disturbance that is characteristic of some types of migration defines vulnerability to HIV, not the origin or the destination of movement" (Decosas et al., 1997). This suggests that the issue of migration and HIV is very complicated, and that in order to comprehend how the two are related, we must take into account the social factors that put migrants at risk for contracting HIV as a result of their reactions to particular socioeconomic conditions in their destinations. Therefore, it is worthwhile to carry out a study of this kind to investigate whether livelihoods, as a socioeconomic element, link to the HIV infection of migrant population, especially those who are living in informal settlements.

Brummer (2002) provided context for the HIV/AIDS epidemic in Southern Africa and argued that environmental variables are what predispose migrants to HIV infection. Given that some migrants settle in urban informal settlements while others do so in urban informal settlements with extremely limited access to amenities, this is likely to be influenced by the environmental circumstances in which immigrants find themselves in their host nations. The risk scenarios, on the other hand, are described by Decosas et al. (1995) as "socially and geographically defined zones where the individual's capacity to respond effectively to a health hazard is limited." Because these reasons prevent migrants from making other choices, their health and welfare are less important, as long as they are making a living.

There is consensus that migrant social, economic, and political marginalization increases migrant vulnerability to HIV (Rijks, 2006). In other words, the sometimes-severe circumstances that migrants encounter, such as poverty, substandard housing, unemployment, and marginalization, increase their sensitivity to HIV infection (Williamson, 2004). To give an example, Peltzer (2003) demonstrates that sex for money or products is frequently employed by women as a survival tactic in situations of acute poverty. On the other hand, because of economic necessity and gender-related expectations that men serve as the family's primary provider, men are compelled to relocate without their families in search of employment. This encourages many sexual interactions, which raises the risk of HIV (Abdool Karim, 2008). The research thus reflects the emerging consensus that a population's susceptibility to infection increases with how socially and economically marginalized it is (Altman, 2005). A word of caution: The association between migration and HIV risk should not be used as justification for blaming migrants for the spread of HIV. Lazarus (2007) noted that risk is a statement about societal situations rather than specific individuals. In other words, rather than being at risk of HIV because of who they are as people, migrants are at risk because of the social and economic marginalization they experience.

Rijks (2006) discovered that people in KwaZulu-Natal were three times more likely to be HIV-positive than those who had lived there their entire lives if they had recently moved or changed dwellings. The higher propensity of migrants to participate in risky activities, such as having multiple sexual partners at their new places, was attributed to the difference in risk. Other research suggests that returning male migrants in rural areas might get HIV through their local female companions. Lurie et al. (2003) demonstrated that HIV can spread from women to their migrant partners, as well as from migrant males returning to their rural partners, in their study on HIV-1 concordance and discordance among migrant and non-migrant couples in South Africa.

PERCEPTION OF HIV RISK, LEVEL OF PRECAUTION, AND BEHAVIOR CHANGE

A sensation of vulnerability or sensitivity to a perceived threat has been described as perception, a cognitive and emotive process that is thought to be a key factor influencing the desire to refrain from risky behavior or engage in self-protective behavior. The problem is that perception is a social and psychological construct that changes depending on the context in which people find themselves. This study describes perception as a means of comprehending concerns that a person has about a particular occurrence, in this case, HIV/AIDS, and the methods a person uses to prevent becoming infected (Adih & Alexandra, 1999). Young males in Ghana were up to six times more likely to use condoms than nonusers if they believed they were in danger of infection (Adih and Alexandra, 1999). However, some research shows the opposing side, that people who do not believe they are at risk of catching the virus were less likely to use condoms. This shows that emphasizing one's vulnerability to HIV infection may not always be sufficient to encourage condom use (Najjumba et al., 2002).

According to Rosenstock (1988), all living things must be able to perceive and escape hazardous environmental situations to survive. He asserted that the capacity to codify and draw lessons from the past is helpful for survival. Humans possess a further ability that enables them to both change and react to their surroundings. This capability increases and decreases risk. The health belief model, as put forth by Rosenstock (1988), contends that an individual's capacity for self-protection or ability to reduce their risk should be influenced by the degree to which they perceive their susceptibility to developing HIV. Despite their perception of risk, a person's desire for protected sex dictates their actions. In light of this, how one feels about using condoms for self-preservation becomes crucial when taking risk perception into account. For instance, given that there are several reasons why women have sex, migrant women's desire for sex generally may influence whether or not they utilize protection. It is important to consider both this and the possibility that not all migrant women may engage in safe sex since some evidence suggests that migrant women who are experiencing hardships may be forced to engage in transactional sex (Adih & Alexandra, 1999).

To be prevented, HIV transmission must be halted before it reaches the human body. The key to doing this is behavior modification (Fan et al., 2007). People must refrain from actions that increase their chance of interaction with the virus to keep the virus from entering their bodies. To prevent the spread of HIV, a great deal of work has been put into studying this area of health behavior modification, particularly in identifying the variables that make people resistant to such changes in their behavior. To highlight key components in modifying health behavior, researchers in the domains of disease prevention and health promotion have arranged their findings in this regard into several models (Fan et al., 2007). The theory of reasoned action and the health belief model (HBM) are two examples of these models (Ogden, 2004).

SOCIOECONOMIC PREDICTORS OF IMMIGRANTS' SEXUAL AND REPRODUCTIVE HEALTH PRODUCT USE

The socioeconomic profile of the community in which a person lives and that person's socioeconomic position both affect that person's risk of contracting HIV. Since HIV infection has been established as one of the non-biological drivers of the epidemic, socioeconomic inequality fosters its spread. The socioeconomic indicators of income, education, and employment status have an impact on a person's risk of contracting HIV (UNAIDS, 2008).

The threat of HIV/AIDS appears less urgent because the poor are more likely to contract the disease because they confront greater hazards in their daily lives. They might not take the necessary precautions to avoid infection as a result. People living in poverty are also less likely to comprehend what AIDS is and how HIV spreads since they have lower levels of education. This assertion is supported by another study that demonstrates a higher HIV prevalence level in the unemployed and unskilled or semi-skilled group. Given that skill levels are likely to be correlated with income levels, low HIV prevalence may therefore be expected at high-income levels. A person's ability to avoid HIV infection and their ability to find sexual partners are both influenced by their socioeconomic status. While males may be able to pay for sex when their income rises, poor women, on the other hand, engage in sex to survive or take on more partners for financial assistance owing to their dire economic situations, thus exposing themselves to HIV infection (UNAIDS, 2008). The level of conflict, level of urbanization, and migration in the community, on the other hand, are related to its socioeconomic profile. Migration promotes the rapid spread of HIV infection and expands the scope of social networking.

Migrants and migrant workers are at an increased risk of contracting HIV since migratory labor has been demonstrated to be closely connected with high-risk sexual behavior. According to research conducted among migrant workers in Carletonville, South Africa, over 50 percent of the male migrant workers had at least one casual partner the previous year. In comparison, 53 percent of the women admitted to taking money for sex. Additionally, it has been discovered that migrants in Carltonville have a higher HIV prevalence rate than non-migrants (Gupta, 2000). According to research, women's economic fragility makes it more likely that they will engage in commercial or transactional sex, and this makes it harder for them to negotiate safety precautions like the use of condoms (Gupta, 2000).

For instance, due to a lack of career possibilities and poor pay, women in Botswana have been economically dependent on men. Because of their vulnerability, women have had a harder time negotiating safer sex or ending dangerous relationships out of fear of becoming destitute in the future (UNAIDS, 2008).

HEALTH BELIEF PREDICTORS OF IMMIGRANTS' CONDOM USE

The health belief model identifies three key factors that explain why there has been little change in health behavior (Fan et al., 2007). The individual's sensitivity to a health risk, such as HIV, is the first factor. The model states that if a person does not think they are in danger of catching a disease, they will not take steps to protect themselves from getting the condition (Ogden, 2004). An individual's perception of the threat posed by the disease is the second significant factor in the health belief model. There is little incentive to take precautionary measures if a person believes that a disease is mild or only poses a little threat. Therefore, to take action to protect oneself against HIV, it is crucial that the person recognizes, understands, and accepts the seriousness of HIV. The third factor is a person's assessment of the success of advised disease prevention measures, such as using condoms as an example. According to the model, it is simpler for a person to decide to take action if the advised course of action is obvious to be effective. The health belief model suggests that perceived severity, susceptibility, and action evaluation are critical elements in changing health behavior (Fan et al., 2007).

CONCLUSION

Most notably for the spread of HIV, migration is frequently linked to a variety of public health issues. It has been observed that women's dependence on men, as well as economic weakness, has increased their susceptibility to HIV by limiting their ability to negotiate condom use. Some men believe that it is against their culture to wear condoms and refuse to do so. The health belief model examined people's actions on the value of using condoms. People must feel intimidated by their present behavior patterns, believe that their health is in danger, and have confidence in their ability to overcome obstacles in order to successfully change their behavior.

REFERENCES

Abdool Karim, Q. (2008). Heterosexual transmission of HIV—the importance of gendered perspective in HIV prevention. In S.S. Abdool Karim & Q. Abdool Karim (Eds.), *HIV/AIDS in South Africa.* New York: Cambridge, 243–61.

Adih, W., & Alexandra, D. (1999). Determinants of condom use to prevent HIV infection among youth in Ghana. *Journal of Adolescent Health* 24: 62–69.

Altman, D. (2005). Rights matter: Structural interventions and vulnerable communities. *Health and Human Rights*, 8(2), 203–13.

Azjen, I. (1991). The theory of planned behavior. *Organizational Behavior and Human Decision Processes*, 50: 179–211.

Bletzer, K. (1995). Use of ethnography in the evaluation and targeting of HIV/AIDS education among Latino farm workers. *AIDS education and prevention* 7(2), 78–91.

Bogart, L.M., Cecil, H., & Pinkerton, S. D. (2000). Hispanic adults' beliefs, attitudes, and intentions regarding the female condom. *Journal of Behavioural Medicine*, 23, 181–206.

Bond, V., & Dover, P. (1997). Men, women and the trouble with condoms: Problems associated with condom use by migrant workers in rural Zambia. *Health Transition* review 7: 377–91.

Brummer, D. (2002). *Labour Migration and HIV/AIDS in Southern Africa.* South Africa: IOM.

Campbell, C. (2000). Selling sex in a time of AIDS: The psycho-social context of condom use by sex workers on a South African mine. *Social Science and Medicine*, 50: 479–94.

Campbell, C. (2003). "Letting them die": *Why HIV/AIDS prevention programmes fail.* Indiana: Indiana University Press.

Decosas, J., & Adrien, A. (1997). *Migration and HIV. AIDS*, 11 (suppl A): S77–S84.

Fan, H. Y., Conner, R. F., & Villarreal, L. P. (2007). *AIDS: Science and society* (5th). Boston: Jones and Bartlett.

Godin, G., et al. (1996). Cross-cultural testing of three social cognitive theories: An application to condom use. *Journal of Applied Social Psychology*, 26: 1556–86.

Gupta, G. D. (2000). Gender, sexuality, and HIV/AIDS: The what, the why and the how. *Canadian HIV/AIDS Policy Law Review*, 5(4): 86–93.

He, N., Detels, R., Zhu, J., Chen, Z., Fang, Y., Zhang, X. et al. (2005). Characteristics and sexually transmitted diseases of male rural migrants in a metropolitan area of Eastern China. *Sexually Transmitted Diseases* 32: 286–92.

International Organization for Migration. (2008). Southern African Migration Project: *HIV/AIDS, Population Mobility, and Migration in Southern Africa: Defining a Research and Policy Agenda.* Geneva: IOM.

IOM. (2005). *HIV/AIDS, population, mobility and migration in Southern Africa.* Geneva: International Organization for Migration.

Kelly, R.J., Gray, R.H., Sewankambo, N.K., Serwadda, D., Wabwire-Mangen, F., Lutalo T. W. (2003). *Age Differences in Sexual Partners and Risk of HIV-1 Infection of Acquired Immune Deficiency Syndromes*, 32(4): 446–51, April 1.

Lazarus, S. (2007). Assumptions and values of community psychology. In N. Duncan, B. Bowman, A. Naidoo, J. Pillay & V. Roos (Eds.). *Community psychology. Analysis, context, and action* (pp. 67–84). Cape Town: UCT Press.

Lurie, M., Harrison, A., Wilkinson, D., Abdool Karim, S.S. (1997). Circular migration and sexual networking in rural Kwazulu Natal: Implications for the spread of HIV and other sexually transmitted diseases. *Health Transition review*. Supp. 3, 15–24.

Lurie, M. N., Williams, B. G., Zuma, K., Mkaya-Mwamburi, D., Garnett, G. P., & Sturm, A. W. (2003, February). The impact of migration on HIV-1 transmission in South Africa. *Sexually Transmitted Diseases*, 30(2): 149–50.

Najjumba, M., Ntozi, J., Ahimbishe, F.E., Odwee, J., Ayiga, N. (2002). Risk perception and condom use in Uganda. *African Population Studies*, 19: 67–80.

Ogden, J. (2004). *Health psychology: A textbook* (3rd ed.). New York: McGraw-Hill.

Peltzer, K. (2003). HIV/AIDS/STD knowledge, attitudes, beliefs and behaviors in a rural South African adult population. *South African Journal of Psychology*, 33(4): 250.

Pfarrwaller, E., & Suris, J.C. (2012). Determinants of health in recently arrived young migrants and refugees: A review of the literature. *Italian Journal of Public Health,* 9(3). Doi: http://dx.Doi.org/10.2427/7529.

Rijks, B. (2006, March). *New partnerships on HIV/AIDS and mobile populations.* Crossings, 7(1), 12. Retrieved February 24, 2008, from http://www.queensu.ca/samp.

Rosenstock, I. (1988). Social learning theory and the health belief model. *Health Education Quarterly,* 15: 175–83.

Salabarria-Pena, Y., Lee, J.W., Montgomery, S. et al. (2003). Determinants of female and male condom use among immigrant women of Central American Descent. *AIDS and Behaviour*, 163–74.

Smith-Estelle, A., & Gruskin, S. (2003). Vulnerability to HIV/STIs among rural women from migrant communities in Nepal: A health and human rights framework. *Reproductive Health Matters,* 11: 142–51.

Tranos, E., Gheasi, M., & Nijkamp, P. (2015). International migration: a global complex network. *Environment and Planning B: Planning and Design*, 42(1): 4–22.

UNAIDS. (2005). *UNAIDS/WHO Epidemiological Fact Sheet—2004 Update*. Retrieved March 2006, from http://www.unaids.org/publications/.

UNAIDS. (2007, December2007 *AIDS epidemic update*. Retrieved February 5, 2008, from http://www.unaids.org/publications.

UNAIDS. (2008). Addressing the societal causes of HIV risk and vulnerability. In *Report on the global AIDS epidemic 2008* (3). Retrieved November 19, 2008, from http://www.unaids.org/en/KnowledgeCentre/HIVData/GlobalReport/2008/2008_Global_report.asp.

Voeten, H. A., Vissers, D. C., Gregson, S., Zaba, B., White, R. G., de Vlas, S. J., & Habbema, J. D. F. (2010). Strong association between in-migration and HIV prevalence in urban sub-Saharan Africa. *Sexually transmitted diseases*, 37(4): 240–43.

Williamson, K. (2004). *AIDS, gender and refugee protection framework.* Oxford: Refugees Studies Centre, University of Oxford.

Yang, X. (2004). Temporary Migration and HIV Risky behaviors: A case study in South Western China. *International Migration Review*, 212–35.

Zuma, K., Gouws, E., Williams, B., & Lurie, M. (2003). Risk factors for HIV infection among women in Carletonville, South Africa: Migration, demography and sexually transmitted diseases. *International Journal of STDs and AIDS* 14, 814–17.

Chapter 7

Home Management of Malaria for Under-Five Children by Migrant Mothers Resident in the Akinyele Local Government Area of Ibadan, Nigeria

Nsere L. Danbagai and
Olufunke Olufunsho Adegoke

INTRODUCTION

The early childhood period is considered the most important developmental phase in an individual's lifespan (Elgibaly and Aziz, 2016). Children under five years of age are particularly vulnerable, accounting for 70 percent of all malaria deaths (United Nations News, 2016), and sub-Saharan Africa carries an excessive share of the global malaria burden. In 2015, the region was an abode of 90 percent of malaria cases and 92 percent of malaria deaths (Olugbade, Isreal, Adedire, Ladipo, Adedokun, Ajumobi, Olayinka, and Ajayi, 2014).

Malaria particularly affects people in tropical and subtropical regions of the world. It remains the most complex and disturbing health problem facing humanity (United Nations News, 2016). It is a severe problem in Africa, due to the favorable conditions for the development of mosquitoes (WHO, 2017). Africa has a very young population; the birth rate is high across most parts of the continent, and in many African countries, more than 40 percent of the population is under fifteen years of age (Worldwide Anti-Malaria Resistance Network, 2018). Given that young children are at higher risk of malaria than adults, this also increases the burden of malaria in Africa compared to other parts of the world. The WHO, in a report, said the number of malaria cases rose in many countries in 2016, suggesting that progress has deteriorated in the global fight against the disease. Nigeria is one of the first three African countries to record an increase in malaria cases of up to five hundred thousand in 2016 (*The Guardian*, 2017).

Access to health care and malaria-control interventions in Africa has been plagued by more general issues of slow development. While national health systems are slowly emerging, many countries are still dependent on foreign aids and NGOs to provide even basic health services. Where these organisations can provide health care, they often face challenges, such as reaching remote residents without good road access, inadequate health professionals, poor medical services, as a result of unreliable electricity or communications networks, and the inability of maintaining supply chains of diagnostic tools and crucial medicine (Worldwide Anti-Malaria Resistance Network, 2018). According to Umar (2012), factors such as distance from home, poverty, the demands of domestic life, perceived low quality of services, drug stock-outs, and the attitude of health workers, amongst others, have led to inconsistent utilization or the bypassing of public health-care facilities.

The status of migrants has also been a strong determinant of mothers' health-seeking behavior. Dang et al. (2018) reported that undocumented migrants rationalise their choice of health-seeking behavior for fear of easy identification by authorities. Prompt diagnosis of children with malaria can help to reduce the rate of death being caused by the ailment. The effective management of malaria upon the discovery of some of the symptoms earlier mentioned can help to curb this trend of malaria killing large numbers of people (WHO, 2017). Quick consultation and early commencement of treatment are proactive ways to combat malaria as early administration of the right medication will help to subdue or even kill the deadly malaria parasite. Also, the issue of the availability of good medical facilities cannot be downplayed to halt this ailment (Malaria Operational Plan, 2017).

In choosing treatment for malaria, factors like perceived and actual quality of care, the proximity of services, accessibility and cost of treatment, socio-economic status of the patients, availability of services, etc., are important. These factors on many occasions constitute constraints that, in turn, make choices explicit, and then patients make compromises between alternatives. Culture also plays an important role in influencing illness recognition and choice of care (Panchi, 2015). Also, social and economic factors that contribute to the appearance of urban malaria are similar to those involved in producing malaria in rural populations and migrants. Hence, settlers on the periphery of urban and semi-urban areas, where malaria commonly occurs, are usually populated by migrants (Adelekan, 2016). Many migrants work parts of the year in the city as wage labourers, and then they return to the country.

People's perceptions and level of knowledge about the cause and mode of transmission of malaria are strong determinants of the preventive measures and health-seeking behaviors to be adopted in combating malaria (Salami and Umego, 2018). Factors such as socioeconomic determinants influence where people and communities live, the kind of environment they live in, how they are treated by others, the goods and services they can provide for themselves, and what society can provide for them (Win, Mung, Waiting, Oo, Thi, Tipmontree, Soonthornworasiri, Kengganpanich, and Kaewkungwal, 2017).

It has been recognized that, in endemic countries, most malaria episodes are treated outside public health facilities, mainly at home (Umar, 2012). Also, environmental hygiene poses an important risk factor in breeding malaria-causing vectors, which will eventually result in people suffering from the malaria disease. Practices such as open drainage systems, lack of disposal system of sewage and solid waste, water stagnation, canal irrigation, animal sheds, increased building constructions, stagnant water, and bushes are factors that aid in the breeding of mosquitoes around the home (Salami and Umego, 2018).

According to Vibrant Health Family (2017), women are the heart of the family. They are also the undisputed family health-care decision-makers, making approximately 80 percent of family health-care decisions. Mothers also choose their children's doctors (85 percent), take them to appointments (84 percent), and ensure they get the recommended care (79 percent) (Kaiser Family Foundation Report, 2018). Invariably, they are the researchers, networkers, and active care advocates, which makes them better able to manage their children's health than the fathers. Home management of malaria, to a large extent, may be void of scientific care delivery (in a hospital), which needs to be looked into to identify how effective and efficient management of malaria is at home.

This study looked at the home management of malaria parasite infections among International migrant mothers with children under five in the Akinyele local government area of Ibadan, Oyo state. The Akinleye local government area of Ibadan is characterized by the presence of a large number of migrants, a poor environment in terms of hygiene and housing, and a high population density, which makes it ideal for research work. Research has shown studies carried out on the management of malaria by mothers with children under five (Kwabe, Abdulfatai, Agbam, and Bashiru, 2013). Also, a review of literature points to several studies that cover the effects of mobility dynamics on socioeconomic behaviors related to malaria control and the choices of a treatment regimen adopted for interventions. Despite the achievements and significant efforts employed by international and national aids in the control of malaria over decades, one major issue that has not been given due consideration is the issue of malaria control in association with international migrant mothers. Little has also been done on how these migrants access early diagnosis and treatments, including their health-seeking behaviors in terms of malaria prevention and management strategies. Little has also been documented about the relationship between their migration status and their health-seeking behaviors. This study, therefore, investigated how migrant mothers with children under the age of five manage malaria in their host communities, considering the different biomes and ecology and how effective these health behaviors are in the management of malaria. Therefore, the study objectives aimed to find out respondents' knowledge, perception, existing social relations, and influencing choice of health-seeking behavior on HMM.

CONCEPTUALIZING MARGINALIZATION

Marginalization is considered a multilayered concept that brings to mind the notion of deprivation resulting from social, economic, and political exclusions that are consequential, especially in relation to the total well-being of an individual or a group irrespective of the geographical location of residence. Marginal experiences can occur in urban, semi-urban, and rural communities. Hence, societies can be marginalized at a global level, in ethnic groups, in families, and at the individual level. The experience of marginality has over decades impacted the lives of millions globally, of which Nigeria is very much included. However, these phenomena are most peculiar to rural and semi-urban dwellers who are challenged by scarce resources. As such, marginals experience poverty, unemployment, discrimination, oppression, and other forms of exclusion, leaving them at a disadvantage. Amongst such categories of marginalized persons are the underprivileged, the exploited, internally displaced persons, and immigrants, amongst others. Nevertheless, marginal experiences are unstable, resulting from natural processes of life changes.

International migrants, by virtue of their migration status, are placed at a disadvantage in host communities. According to empirical studies carried out on migrants, a large number of migrants reside in rural and semi-urban areas that are economically deprived, with scarce resources and opportunities. Such communities are categorically slummed, with an unhealthy physical environment characterised by dilapidated structures, thick bushes, the presence of dirty, stagnant water, poor drainage systems, poor waste management systems, bad roads, poor access to health-care services, and a lack of other basic amenities, amongst others. Furthermore, these international migrants, according to the literature, are largely undocumented, hence they are disadvantaged at getting highly paid economic jobs or having the ability to reside in urban communities for fear of identification and harassment by the government resulting from their illegal status in the country. Hence, they are saddled with the option of hiding in communities with less government attention and economic opportunities. Thus, international migrant residents at the Akinyele local government area of Ibadan, Oyo state, are very much included in those experiencing marginalization.

THEORETICAL THRUST

The health belief model (HBM) is a value expectancy theory that health actions available to an individual would prevent undesirable consequences (Tarkang and Zotor, 2015). It looks at health-seeking behaviors by highlighting that which enable or prevent people from making "healthy choices," in either their lifestyle behaviors or their use of medical care and treatment. HBM responds specifically to knowledge and perceived ill health. Health-promoting behaviors are adopted based on a mixture of demographic, social, emotional, and cognitive factors, perceived symptoms, access to care, and personality. The underlying assumption is that behaviors are best understood in terms of the knowledge and perception of the social environment. This theory assumes that those who believe they have control over their health are more likely to engage in health-promoting behaviors.

Furthermore, the HBM's attempts to predict health behaviors through a variety of means is predicated on two assumptions central to classic health promotion: first, that health is influenced by behaviors, and second, that behaviors are modifiable. Therefore, it perceives people as rational decision-makers, systematically reviewing the available information and forming behaviors and intentions. It is recognized that these factors could influence the behaviors of individuals and therefore are crucial in health-promotion practices.

The basics of this theory are to assess health behaviors through an understanding of knowledge, perceptions, and attitudes people have towards disease and its outcomes, especially negative outcomes. It also sets out to motivate caregivers to take proper actions to avoid these negative health outcomes being "rational beings." Hence, the health belief model points out that perceptions are formed around the quality and efficient health information available to these international migrant mothers, which, in turn, impacts the health outcomes of the children under the age of five, and their families at large. Therefore, it is apt to say that these international migrant mothers develop their health-seeking behaviors according to their rationality of what they perceive to be right for them, their younger children, and the family in its entirety. These actions were moulded from the quality and quantity of information they gathered as it concerns malaria disease, including other socio-cultural factors, such as experiences, personal beliefs, religious beliefs, etc.

METHODOLOGY

This was an ethnographic study that employed an explorative research design. The qualitative research technique involved the use of key informant interviews (KII), in-depth interviews (IDI), and the observation method, which identified the relationship between their social and behavioral patterns as it affects or influences their home management of malaria (HMM) in the Akinyele local government area of Ibadan, Oyo state. The target population for this study consisted of international migrant mothers who have children between the age ranges of zero to five years. These international migrant mothers are nationals from Ghana, Togo, Chad, Senegal, Mali, Gambia, Guinea, and Sierra Leone. Also included were their spouses and the community health-care workers residing in the Akinyele local government area of Ibadan. The sample size for this study was twenty participants selected from the international migrants and the health-care workers These participants were purposefully selected representatively across the communities (Ojoo, Sasa, and Moniya) identified as hubs of these international migrants in Akinyele, LGA. The research instruments for the study were in-depth interviews and key informant interview guides. The observation technique was also deployed in the process of data collection with a focus on the environment and cultural life of the participants. Analysis of the data was done thematically guided by the research questions. Consent was sought from the participants before engaging them in the participation of the study. All ethical principles of confidentiality, beneficence, and justice was adhered to.

RESULTS

Socio-Demographic Information of Respondents

The socio-demographic characteristics have to do with the social and demographic characteristics of the respondents, which included age, marital status, nationality, religion, number of years in residing in Nigeria, level of education, occupation, level of income, marriage type, number of children, number of children below the ages of five, and migration status. The demographic distribution of these participant migrants according to age ranged from twenty-four to sixty-five years. These were international migrants from other African counties, namely Ghana, Togo, Chad, Senegal, Mali, Gambia,

Guinea, and Sierra Leone. These migrants are mostly of the Islam faith with an Islamic education. Also, they are largely traders or housewives with an income of less than N18,000.00. Their spouses are artisans and miners.

Respondents' Knowledge on Home Management of Malaria for Children Under Five

Investigation revealed the international migrants' knowledge of malaria as a sickness from mosquito bite, with the indication of signs and symptoms to include fever, vomiting, loss of appetite, high temperature, fatigue, and weakness, and indicated fever and cold. The malaria disease is transmitted through the bite of the mosquito. The International Migrant Mothers commonly termed *malaria* as "Beri-Beri" or "yellow fever." They also assert that malaria is a trigger for other health conditions, such as typhoid, cholera, and diarrhoea. As stated by a respondent:

> It is sickness from mosquito bite. Look, any other sickness does not surface until there is mosquito bite . . . so we can even say that mosquito bite can lead to typhoid and diarrhoea. (IDI/Female/Muslim/47/Arabic studies/Togolese/Sasa/2020).

Other research respondents confirmed by stating that:

> We call it Beri-Beri. It is yellow fever . . . Yellow fever is malaria. It is sickness from mosquito bite. That is what we know it to be. Also, it is the major illness we suffer from in this community. Our children are not even left out. Just take a look at this community. We have every reason to fall sick. Look around, this community is very dirty from bushes around, and dirty drainage. Tell the government on our behalf to come and help we the poor people. (IDI/Female/Muslim/39/Arabic studies/Niger/Sasa/2020)

Based on this study, the role played by environmental hygiene cannot be overemphasized. Environmental hygiene poses a great threat to the stability of human life, especially to the children who have weak immune systems. The hygiene practices include the construction of proper drainage systems, proper waste management system, improved housing construction, cleaning up the environment such as cutting down bushes, proper sewage management, and many more. Based on the data collected, international migrant mothers are quite knowledgeable about the adverse effects that poor hygiene practices and behaviors affect have on the stability of their health and that of their family members, especially the children under the age of five. According to a key informant interview with a community health-care worker:

> The migrants know their environment causes malaria. Although they might be able to identify the signs and symptoms of malaria, they don't always know what the sign is saying. The child might be having an ordinary headache from stress and not malaria. So, their knowledge is not adequate as regards malaria. This does not mean that they don't know anything, because we try to educate them about their health, especially the mothers when they come for antenatal visits and the children's clinic. It is actually not easy to communicate with all of them, because not all of them understand English and Yoruba, which is an alternative language for communicating with them. (KII/CHW/female/2 years in LGA/Ojoo PHC/2020)

Furthermore, respondents are knowledgeable about mosquito habitats around their house by indicating stagnant water, bushes, dirty places, poor drainage system, and poor toilet maintenance. This shows that the community under study, based on data collected and observation, is bushy, has lots of stagnant water, and has a very dirty environment with a very bad drainage system. This invariably provides the conditions necessary to increase the chances of mosquitoes, with the respondents clearly stating the presence of water, rainfall, bushes, and warm temperatures to be the perfect breeding environment for mosquitos' parasites, with the rainy season most suitable for the breeding of mosquitoes. Children during this season, as reported by the respondents, have more episodes of malaria at this time of the year, especially at night.

Also, the respondents seem to have heard about malaria and its preventive and management strategies, with a small number of them never hearing about it with personally discovering these measures through various mediums such as from friends/family, radio, television, and the internet. It is evident these international migrants have all it takes to be enlightened about malaria. The knowledge of a phenomena is key to being able to address it and proffer suitable solutions. Based on the findings of this research work, these mothers confirmed their level of awareness via different communication mediums by which they get informed.

As regards this, this is what a respondent had to say:

> This mosquito mostly lives inside water . . . Not just water, it is those dirty waters beside the road . . . Like inside the gutter. Water that is not moving. And when rain fall again, mosquito go increase because you know say they need water to make them survive and increase too. And anywhere where it is dirty, you must find them there. We know and we suppose they clean our environment. (IDI/Female/Muslim/51/Primary/Senegalese/Sasa/2020)

Hence, as knowledgeable as these international migrants are, based on the research findings, not all of them actually apply the acquired knowledge due to some subjective reasons, such as having the feeling of being cheated for individually engaging in environmental hygiene, which should be a community responsibility. Irrespective of some communication barriers, such as language and literacy level, these mothers have not been isolated in acquiring the necessary knowledge needed to pull them through their desire to maintain stable health conditions for them and their families, especially that of their younger children. Some of these mediums include radio, television, and health education by health workers, especially during special days for the children's clinic. Friends and family have also played very key roles in their knowledge acquisition, as they share ideas amongst themselves as regards the measure to put in place that will efficiently manage the disease. This could also be achieved by mere observing other female neighbours since their homes are closely knitted. A respondent had this to say as regards to the source of information:

> Una (your) government they no try for we the migrants. They don't even provide us with things that we need. We always hear am for radio say them don't send mosquito-treated nets to us, but we no see anything. Then go bring am plenty for inside trailer, then go they sell am like N100 or N200. We know they say this is supposed to be free, but we no know why then they sell am. (IDI/Female/Muslim/43/None/Togolese/Sasa/2020)

The role of the government in combating malaria cannot be overemphasized. From research, the government has made efforts to be of assistance to the masses, especially as regards their health, thereby providing free-insecticide treated nets, subsidized treatment rates, subsidized cost of drugs, and free health education and awareness. According to the study, some respondents acknowledged that the government has been putting resounding efforts forth to assist the masses, but they identified that despite these efforts, the beneficiaries do not actually benefit from these government-assistance schemes. Some respondents specifically identified that this insecticide-treated nets are being sold to them at the rate of N100 or N200, which goes against the original motive for the assistance. Furthermore, a health-care worker had this to say:

> Many of these women frequently report that their children have malaria because they don't take good care of their environment. If you go there, you will see a lot of stagnant water, breeding mosquito empires that will subsequently bite the child who does not have a strong immune system yet against malaria. Measures have been put in place to address their health needs. For example, the government has tried to distribute free insecticide nets to them and free drugs. All they have to do is bring their children to the hospital for proper treatment; all they have to do is give a little token to get a file that covers them and their family members. Policies have also been put in place by the government to

> address the management of malaria. The policy covers the use of ACT, which is artemisinin-based combined test, and RDT, which means rapid diagnostic test, to first diagnose the patient and confirm the ailment before administering treatments so as not to administer the wrong treatment, which may result in increased health conditions or even loss of life at worse. (KII/Doctor/male/20 years in LGA/Moniya/2020)

Artesunate combination therapy (ACT) and rapid diagnostic therapy (RDT) as malaria-health policies covers the procedure of treatment, the cost, the drugs' availability, and compliance level amongst mothers. Furthermore, for children's protection against contracting malaria, the majority of the respondents praised the usage of mosquito nets, ensuring a clean environment, repellent, regular shutting of windows and doors, and usage of insecticides. These are significant strategies for managing malaria. A respondent had this to say:

> My children have had episodes of malaria, but it is not often. They fall sick once in a while. We know how bad malaria can be. We know what causes it. We know what to do so that our children will not be falling sick again. We too as parents will rest from spending so much money to treat them. Like me now, since I know that mosquitos like to be where there is water whether it is clean or not . . . Ah, they are clean animals so if the water is not covered, they will be there. So, I have made sure that my wife bought covers for all our water, and once there is water on the floor, it must be cleaned so they will not have that room to come and stay. I even made sure I put nets on every window and door so that we can leave the door open if there is heat and for ventilation. So, how can they fall sick? And my wife is not a dirty woman; she tries really hard to make sure she keeps the house very clean. (KII/Male/Muslim/49/Ghanaian/Sasa/2020)

In addition, treatment options in managing malaria range from over-the-counter drugs serving as a first point of treatment option as identified by of the respondent. Other treatment options include consulting with health professionals, indicated use of herbs, indicated personal hygiene, while other respondents combine these management strategies. This includes the usage of over-the-counter drugs and the use of herbs, the use of herbs and consultation with professionals, and the combination of over-the-counter drugs and consultation with professionals. From these results, in as much as over-the-counter drugs are mostly used, professional health-care services have equal significance, including the use of herbs.

Finally, it is shown that almost all of the respondents indicated the usage of mosquito nets as a preventive measure for protecting the children from mosquitos, indicated ensuring a clean environment, indicated the use of insecticides, indicated both ensuring a clean environment and the use of insecticide, indicated the use of mosquito repellent, signified the use of herbs, signified that they do not have an idea, while others indicated the regular closure of doors/windows. Based on this study, the use of insecticide-treated nets has been identified by the respondents to be the best preventive measure of malaria. According to a respondent:

> We use to clean out environment every time. In fact, we wash the toilet every day so that mosquitos will not build a house with us and affect my small child. (IDI/Female/Christian/primary/38/Gambian/Sasa/2020)

Another respondent also stated this:

> We put on mosquito coil at least three times in a week because of the small children. They are very prone to falling sick once there is slight mosquito bite. Another thing I do is that whether they fall sick or not, I give them herbs constantly, which is meant to prevent them from contacting any sickness, and it has really been of help because my children don't fall sick all the time. It has been working for me this way. (IDI/Female/Muslim/Islamic studies/33/Malian/Sasa/2020)

From this study, the prevention of malaria goes beyond the use of the insecticide-treated net and other hygiene practices. As stated by a respondent, herbs are used to prevent these young children from contracting this disease and other forms of disease by the mothers administering it to their children for consumption as a daily health regiment for the prevention of disease and immune boosting. This, according to the respondent, has been effective in controlling how frequently her children fall ill. Also, a male international migrant, who has been a household member and participant observer, had this to say:

> There are a lot of bushes that surround where we live. So, when it is the rainy season, we make sure we clear the bushes regularly. After clearing the bush, we sometimes get insecticides from the government to kill the growth of the grass again for a long time. (KII/Male/Muslim/BSc/45/Niger/Ojoo/2020)

According to a KII interview, a matron has this to say:

> You see, many of these women do self-drug prescription and administration. Any slight headache, they think it is malaria and just do self-treatment. But I always advise that they should go to the primary health-care centre before taking any drug. Fine, they always take paracetamol, but it is still an over-the-counter drug, which is not supposed to be encouraging. However, we understand that the poor economy causes many of them not to attend the primary health-care centre anyway. We want them to come. The government has tried to subsidize the cost for them. The government can still support in any way(s) they can . . .

in the hospital, we don't care where you come from, whether you are a Nigerian or not, or even if you are a registered migrant or not. What we do is administer treatment if you present yourself and your children. Besides, no one will ask you if you are registered or not. (KII/Doctor/3 years in LGA/Ojoo PHC/2020).

Furthermore, the Nigerian policy on health for all is being synced by the professional health-care givers whom, research has shown, puts the health of individuals, especially the vulnerable groups, into consideration, as every individual has the right to life and sound health. Therefore, this shows that the status of migrants is not a determinant to health for them and their entire household, especially for the younger children.

Respondents' Conduct in the Management of Malaria for Children Under Five

Conducting HMM will involve the interplay of certain activities and health-seeking behaviors. The severity of malaria cannot be sidelined, as this can be a determining factor for the actions these mothers will engage in to care for their children, which can appear as mild, serious, or very serious, with a large number of mothers experiencing the deaths of their children. Home management of malaria as the first call of many mothers indicates that it is an effective health-seeking behavior, with many migrant mothers attesting to it. This has been a first point of call for majority of the mothers before consulting the health-care professional. According to the health-care workers, the health-seeking behaviors of migrant mothers, according to field results, is largely influenced by their socio-demographic characteristics and their socio-cultural orientations relating to health, illness, and illness behaviors, such as age, religion, education, level of income, migration status, personal beliefs, and others. The health-care workers highlights this below:

In managing malaria in children, it is important that the child is made to use the drugs according to how it was prescribed. It is wrong not to complete the dosage of the prescribed drugs. It is also wrong to use it the wrong way. For instance, some always combine prescribed drugs with local herbs. This is not always advisable, as it might cause complications. Also, caregivers should note that when you are asked to use four in the morning and four in the night, it is dangerous to combine everything together in the night. This can cause complications. (KII/Male/Doctor/3 years LGA/PHC Ojoo/2020)

One community health-care worker said:

Once a child is noticed to be having health-challenging signs and symptoms, I always advise that the mother or caregiver should try as much as possible to take

> minimal first aid first, and thereafter bring the child immediately to the clinic. Using over-the-counter drugs is dangerous and can lead to more danger for the health of the children. (KII/Female/CHW/2 years LGA/Ojoo PHC/2020)

Hence, at the first sign of ill health in their children, a large number of the respondents administer over-the-counter drugs as the first course of action, with the majority of the respondents combating the disease at its first signs and symptoms with over-the-counter drugs. Also, after administering first aid to affected children, some of these mothers take a window period of two to four days to observe the condition of the children. In case of slowed or no improvement, the mothers then consult professional help. With regard to this, a respondent said:

> I always feel afraid because the child will suddenly develop high temperature. After that, she will then start to cry, and before you know it, her eyes will turn coloured at night. I cannot speak for other women, but for me, as soon as she starts to show certain signs, like increased temperature, loss of appetite, and I don't see her playing, I will know there is a problem. I will quickly give here paracetamol. It worries me because I know that my baby plays a lot and seeing her all drawn to herself scares me. Also, I personally don't joke around with my children's health. I like them strong. (IDI/Female/ Muslim/36/Guinea / Sasa/2020).

Furthermore, in the administration of first aid for children with malaria episodes, these migrant mothers choose a range of treatment and management options, which includes the utilization of over-the-counter drugs and the use of herbs such as "rai daure," "ganyen lele," and lemongrass, all mixed with lemon. According to a respondent:

> When our children are down with malaria and other sicknesses, we buy drugs from the medicine store and give to them. We also give them herbs like rai daure, ganyen tea, and ganyen lele. We combine these leaves with lemon so it can be effective. We use them to threat malaria and other sicknesses, like typhoid, yellow fever. You should know that these leaves are very medicinal, and they treat a lot of ailments in the body we don't even know about. They will cleanse your whole body. (IDI/Female/Muslim/41/Guinea/Sasa/2020)

This was further confirmed by another respondent, who stated:

> I give my children lemongrass with lemon. We do not have any special herbs we bring from our country of origin. We use what is available to us here. Besides, how much would it cost us to go to our country to bring our own herbs? When your child is sick, people around will tell you to use some leaves, and they will show you and it works. It has been working for us. Also, we don't stop at that;

> we buy medicine from the shop to give them when they fall sick. It is better to combine them. (IDI/Female/Muslim/45/Senegal/Sasa/2020).

According to the respondents, the individual methods they employ have always been effective in controlling malaria for their children and household. Hence, on the average, being parents, the mothers have the best interests of their children at heart, and therefore they will employ strategies they perceive will aid them in giving their wards sound health. It is important to note that, irrespective of this health behavior, it is advantageous to seek professional help as health workers are trained to execute health-care issues.

Factors Influencing Respondents Choice of Home Management of Malaria for Children Under Five

The home management of malaria is determined by certain factors, ranging from socio-cultural and economic factors. The findings revealed that factors such as age, marital status, religion, length of stay in Nigeria, level of education, income level, family type, number of children, and migration status influences home management of malaria. Factors such as religion and level of income have been seen to be of significant influence on the respondent's choice of HMM. Where the cost of regiment is high, mothers will opt for what they can afford. From this study, we see that the majority of the mothers are housewives or they only engage in low-paying businesses, thereby earning below the minimum wage, stipulated to be N18,000 in Nigeria. This can be predicted as such because the more educated the mothers are about the phenomena, the more proactive health behavior will be adopted. Other variables of influence include cultural dispositions, such as personal beliefs, illness perception, and social organization; these are key factors to malaria management.

Furthermore, social relations do influence the choice of HMM among these respondents. The home management of malaria involves a synthesis of social interactions that could be direct, as it is believed that no man is an island on his own. Research findings reveal that some respondents should take immediate action as soon as they perceive any unhealthy behavior or condition. However, a small number of mothers stated they do not take immediate action to care for their children for various reasons, which may include personal convictions as well as the severity of the illness. Also, others wait to take their cue from their spouses. This could be for economic reasons, as the male parents are largely saddled with the responsibility for providing financial support to the family. Religious sentiments attached to a woman being subordinate to the man holds that women should only exercise what the man permits her to do; this may also be a determining factor. One respondent stated that:

> You ask what my role is in assisting my wife care for the children. I am very much involved in the life of my children even though we are not together. I have two wives, one in the north and the other here with me. My wives cannot make any decision without involving me, even if I am far away. I am the one providing the money for the treatments, and so they have to involve me so I can know what I am spending. They will have to put a call through, telling me that my child is not well. Then, I will give those instructions on what to do. I personally prefer them to take the child to the hospital, but sometimes I will ask them to administer paracetamol first and monitor the child. If symptoms remain or become worse, they will inform me, and I will ask them to the take the child to the hospital. The only exception to this, when they take action and later inform me, is when they cannot reach me and the condition needs to be attended to immediately after administering first aid. Even my religion does not permit women to do as they please, as they are under their husbands. (KII/Male/Muslim/47/Niger/Sasa/2020)

In addition, a majority of the mothers have had direct or indirect relations, which has influenced their malaria management behaviors. According to a respondent:

> I do not need to wait for my husband before I take my child to the hospital. Their health is very important to me. First of all, sometimes as mothers, when you try something out and it is not working, you can ask your friend or neighbour for advice. We share ideas. There is this plant that I was given by my neighbour—it does not only work for malaria, but it works for other sicknesses too. I even give it to my children for preventing illnesses. But ultimately, I take my children to the hospital for proper checkups. I cannot afford to allow them fall ill anyhow. I will do whatever I need to do to keep them healthy. If I don't do it, I myself will suffer too. (IDI/Female/Muslim/Primary/35/Ghanaian/Sasa/2020)

Furthermore, research findings revealed that more of the respondents have supportive friends to consult. As regards this, a large number of these mothers state that their friends are experienced with managing malaria episodes. This may serve as the reason why these mothers consult their friends. Hence, most of the respondents assert that consulting friends has been of great significance to them as the quality of their children's health has been progressive. Therefore, the role of friends in aiding other mothers to care for their younger children cannot be overemphasized. Mothers with children gradually become experienced on effective and efficient preventing and management strategies to employ on varying degrees when they encounter a series of malaria episodes with their children.

Further, according to the field outcome, a large number of these mothers prefer to use traditional methods of care; however, they largely recommend the utilization of a combined method of malaria prevention and management for best results against malaria, which has been very effective and efficient.

Perception of the Home Management of Malaria

It is shown that more of the respondents disagreed that when non-prescribed drugs failed to work, a doctor's advice is not important. Doctors' advice is of great significance irrespective of the failure of prescribed or non-prescribed drugs. The failure of drugs is bounded by factors, such as expiration date or even administering the wrong treatment regimen to children for the consumption void of clinical diagnostics with equivalent treatment options proffered. A large number of these mothers are falling prey to the easy access and affordability of over-the-counter drugs, with more participants not consulting the doctor for all drug prescriptions. Also, an overwhelming proportion of these mothers use previously prescribed drugs when similar symptoms reappeared, or by using old prescriptions to get new drugs. Some mothers perceive symptoms such as fever, headache, vomiting, loss of appetite, and many others to be the symptoms for malaria and only malaria. According to one health worker, various diseases share similar signs and symptoms, with the most common being fever, headache, and vomiting. Therefore, these symptoms do not necessarily translate to malaria. According to a health worker:

> A majority of the women would rather stay at home to administer their own treatment instead of bringing their younger children to the hospital for proper treatment. Once they become aware that their children start to show signs and symptoms, such as fever, headache, vomiting, loss of appetite, and many others, they will just conclude that it is malaria that has affected the child, not knowing that those signs and symptoms they see could be as a result of other illness that is not malaria. In fact, when they come to the health centre, they report malaria as the condition affecting the child, since the child has an increased temperature. This puts the life of the child in jeopardy, as more harm can be done rather than giving recovery. They mostly prefer to bring the child to the hospital when they have tried all other possible solutions and they are not working. They should bring these children here so that they can be tested and treated accordingly. (KII/CHW/Female/2 years in LGA/Ojoo/2020)

Most of these mothers perceive that the administration of herbal medicine to children under five years old is bad. According to a respondent:

> Me I no dey give my pikin "Agbo" o. I no like am. Since my own papa and mama born me, den give me Agbo only one time and e no do well for my body. Me I no go give my pikin o. Den say their own parents no they give them. You know say everybody body different. E get people weh if dem give the Agbo, e

> go work for them pass hospital medicine. As some people dey again weh b say their own body na hospital medicine good for them. Make people dey know wetin good for them before den do am. And again, the problem with this Agbo be say, then no dey fit measure am. Person fit drink pass wetin him suppose dink e go come become problem for am. But for me o, I go talk say e bad for children. If big person wan drink am, I no get problem with am but no b small pikin weh body never strong finish. (IDI/Female/Muslim/Islamic studies/34/Sasa/2020)

Hence, based on the results shown, it is revealed that participants typically indulge in self-medication. This is a considerable statistic to assert that mothers generally indulge in self-medication irrespective of further measures employed. The home management of malaria has been integrated into the health-care system and has been identified to be effective, but only as a point of first aid. According to a respondent:

> Yes, we know that most of these mothers try to manage malaria at home. Some methods have proven to be effective. We are not asking them to stop because some of them do a good job of putting the sickness under control before bringing the child to us here. What we are campaigning for is that, even if they administer any form of treatment, they should bring the child to the hospital for further checkup. (KII/Male/Doctor/14 years in LGA/Sasa PHC/2020)

According to an IDI, a man had this to say in response to the management of malaria at home:

> Well, I do instruct my wife sometimes about what to do when the child shows some signs of malaria. But sincerely, I like how my wives respond to my children anytime they are sick. Oftentimes, they will first call me and tell me that the child is running a temperature. I will then send them to someone to get paracetamol to use for the child first . . . Then they should take the child to the hospital if I am not nearby. Sometimes, my wives use herbs when the temperature is too high for the child. The herbs even prevent the children from having malaria. So, they give it to the children oftentimes. (KII/Male/Muslim/Arabic studies/47/Niger/Sasa/2020)

From research results, it is shown that more of the respondents indicated that they seek help from the hospital for the management of malaria in a child under five years old. Some seek help from the combination of the usage of over-the-counter drugs, herbs, and going to the hospital, while others indicated they did not know how to seek for help. Further, more of the respondents considered affordability, service quality, proximity, personal choice, and other factors, including time, before seeking for care for their children under the age of five.

Finally, respondents, as regards to medicine utilization, largely opined to the combination of alternative and orthodox medicine to care for their children. A key informant interviewee has this to say:

> In managing malaria in children, it is important that the child is made to use the drugs according to how they were prescribed. It is wrong not to complete the dosage of the prescribed drugs. It is also wrong to use them the wrong way. For instance, some always combine prescribed drugs with local herbs. This is not always advisable, as it might cause complications. Also, caregivers should note that when you are asked to use four in the morning and four in the night, it is dangerous to combine everything together in the night. This can cause complications. (KII/Doctor/Male/3 years in LGA/PHC Ojoo/2020)

The community health-care worker said:

> Once a child is noticed to be having health-challenging signs and symptoms, I always advise that the mother or caregiver should try as much as possible to use first aid first, and thereafter bring the child immediately to the clinic. Using over-the-counter drugs is dangerous and can lead to more danger for the health of the children. (KII/CHW/female/2 years in LGA/PHC Ojoo/2020)

Health Seeking Behaviors in the Management of Malaria for Children Under Five

The health-seeking behaviors of migrant mothers according to the field results is largely influenced by their socio-demographic characteristics and socio-cultural orientations relating to health, illness, and illness behaviors, such as age, religion, education, level of income, migration status, personal beliefs, and others.

A key informant interviewee has this to say:

> In managing malaria in children, it is important that the child is made to use the drugs according to how it was prescribed. It is wrong not to complete the dosage of prescribed drugs. It is also wrong to use it the wrong way. For instance, some always combine prescribed drugs with local herbs. This is not always advisable, as it might cause complications. Also, caregivers should note that when you are asked to use four in the morning and four in the night, it is dangerous to combine everything together in the night. This can cause complications. (KII/Male/Doctor/3 years LGA/PHC Ojoo/2020)

The community health-care worker said:

> Once a child is noticed to be having health-challenging signs and symptoms, I always advise that the mother or caregiver should try as much as possible to use

minimal first aid first, and thereafter bring the child immediately to the clinic. Using over-the-counter drugs is dangerous and can lead to more danger for the health of the children. (KII/Female/CHW/2 years LGA/Ojoo PHC/2020)

DISCUSSION OF FINDINGS

The theoretical discussion of findings is discussed within the context of the health belief model and functionalism theory, which emphasises the roles of mothers and their health-seeking behaviors as they concern their children under the age of five. According to the health belief model, mothers are rational beings who engage in certain health-seeking behaviors to either prevent or manage the health of their family members, especially their younger children under the age of five. These behaviors can generate positive or negative outcomes.

Based on the health belief model, the perceived susceptibility of health influenced a person's subjective perception of the chance of contracting a disease, which can be due to the biological makeup of individuals, such as children under the age of five. Children in this age group, according to the Worldwide Anti-Malaria Resistance Network (2018), are very vulnerable to diseases and infections, due to their poorly developed immune systems. The health behavior of these mothers are of great significance in preventing or managing malaria at home. According to the study, results showed that the health behaviors engaged in by these mothers includes the use of insecticide-treated nets and the cleaning of individual rooms. Nevertheless, irrespective of the proactive health behaviors engaged in by these mothers, which covers basically their immediately surroundings (their rooms), the community is falling short in these proactive behaviors. This, the study revealed, is due to the perception of "monkey go work, baboon go chop," as the saying goes in Nigerian pidgin. In essence, these international migrant mothers, according to a KII, would rather clean their rooms than clean the environment for others to benefit from. This is posed to be a non-proactive health behavior, as the total environment affects the well-being of individuals, especially the vulnerable in the community such as younger children under the age of five. Hence, this invariably exposes the children to ill health.

Respondents' knowledge on HMM for children under the age of five revealed that almost all the women have heard of malaria, and they also associate malaria with mosquito bites and unhygienic food items. Also, these international migrant mothers perceive that malaria is a trigger for other health conditions, and it also translates into other conditions such as diarrhoea, cholera, and typhoid. From the study, despite having working knowledge of malaria's signs and symptoms, not all of them could give the vivid signs and symptoms of malaria. Also, it was revealed that when it comes to controlling malaria, an overwhelming proportion of them adopt different or a combination of two or more styles of malaria prevention. All the participants opined that mosquito bites contribute immensely to malaria in their children.

Similarly, a study carried out by Birhanu (2016) revealed that knowledge about the signs and symptoms of malaria was very high, amongst which chills (87.3 percent), fever or a hot body (74.1 percent), and headache (73.1 percent) were the most frequently mentioned signs and symptoms of malaria. The study also revealed that community members often define *malaria illness* in terms of fever, headache, or cold, with loss of appetite. Birhanu et al. (2016), in their work, identified mothers' knowledge of the perceived causes of malaria as being mosquito bite (75 percent) and unhygienic food/drink (43 percent) as the leading causes of malaria.

The study also discovered that mothers adopt various styles in home management against malaria in children under five years of age. Some of the identified means of controlling for the main source, mosquito bite, includes the use of mosquito nets, ensuring clean environment, making sure that windows and doors are always shut, the use of insecticides, the use of mosquito repellent, the use of mosquito coil, or the combination of all these identified means of controlling mosquito bites. Most of the respondents indicated that the chosen mechanism against malaria is usually effective to a reasonable extent.

The study further found there are factors that influence women's choice of home management of malaria. This includes distance from the health-care facility, economic reasons, the time factor, the services rendered at the hospital, among others. However, the majority of the participants indicated that the facilities provided in the health centre are okay, but they didn't always get the best due to the non-availability of adequate drugs. When it comes to service delivery, there seems to be no problem, but for economic reasons, they are oftentimes discouraged.

According to the health belief model, mothers perform certain health behaviors based on what is accessible to them and what serves as barriers to the type and quality of health they deserve and want for their children and family members. The cost of treatment is one of the major factors determining the choice of malaria treatment in Nigeria. It has been a major barrier and determinant of health in Nigeria. Access to ACTs is still constrained by cost, as they cost much more than the previously used anti-malaria drugs, with a dose averaging about 500 naira, (Oladepo, 2008). The high cost of ACTs often results in patients opting for a cheaper alternative or not purchasing the complete regimen. This is further compounded by the lack of financial risk protection in Nigeria, especially for the informal sector, where a large number of the population belong. This means that even the poor people pay out of pocket to receive treatment each time their children have malaria episodes, which could be several times a year. Choice is influenced by prices (including travel and time costs of seeking treatment), income, lack of information about appropriate treatments, and the difficulties patients have in assessing quality treatment.

Cues to actions are triggers to decisions. Based on the research, a large number of the international migrants mothers are Muslims. Based on this study, the results reveal that most of these international migrant mothers take cues from their husbands as to when to access treatment for their children, including the type of treatment to be administered. According to a male KII respondent, this health behavior is due to the fact that the husbands, as heads of the family, are saddled with the responsibility of funding for the family in every aspect, including their health; therefore, they should be involved or informed first before making any decision, as it is not the mother's place to make family decisions unless the roles will be switched with the mothers paying the bills for the family. This invariably poses as a negative health behavior, as children's health may become at risk.

Also, there is an existing social relation in the home management of malaria for children under the age of five, where respondents tend to contact persons with whom they have developed reasonable relationships when the child develops sickness. This could include family members, friends, and community health-care centre professionals, subscribing to both modern and traditional means of treating the sick child. Also, malaria perception, according to these mothers, hinges on the severity, and what the person believes of the sickness, as truly they have at one point or the other subscribed to the usage of drugs that are not prescribed just to save the situation when it comes to an emergency. Some even go to the extent of purchasing a drug that was prescribed in the past to treat malaria. Also, some women indicated that they make use of abandoned drugs to treat malaria, when worse comes to worst on treating malaria. An overwhelming number of respondents agreed that they are guilty of self-medication in treating malaria in children under the age of five.

Kio et al. (2016) asserts that the perception among most parents and caregivers about malaria and its causes has been negative. Most parents and caregivers believe that harmful outcomes result if fever is not treated, irrespective of the severity of malaria. The main concerns among caregivers due to unmanaged fever remain febrile convulsions, damage to the brain, and death, with several cases of malaria in children being managed at home prior to presentation at health-care facilities. This practice of home management of the fever happens to be common among caregivers in Nigeria and other sub-Saharan African countries.

When it comes to health seeking behaviors in the management of malaria for children under the age of five, most women indicated that their first line of action is to buy drugs, whether over-the-counter or prescribed. The majority already had an idea of the signs and symptoms their children display when he/she is about to fall sick. Apart from making the decision first in treating the children, the spouse (husband) tends to be the next person to contact for a decision as regards treating the child. When the husband decides, the next person in line tends to be the community health-care worker(s). There are various reasons that determines their decision, and this includes affordability, personal conviction, the severity of the disease, the level of health awareness, or the combination of all.

In a study carried out on health-seeking behavior and treatment intentions of fever, the home treatment of fever was primarily performed by partially disrobing and exposing children to ambient air, sponging them with tepid water, and using antipyretics, such as paracetamol (Elsinga, 2015). Antimalarial medications and antibiotics were rarely used. In Nigeria, antimalarial medication would have been used by about 71 percent of mothers on their children at home for treatments of fever prior to reporting at health-care facilities (Sangowawa, Amodu, Olaniyan, Amodu, Olumese, and Omotade, 2014). Hence, malaria is often diagnosed based on clients providing an oral history of their children's symptoms.

In essence, the perceived severity of the disease is a cue to action. This has propagated certain health behaviors amongst international migrants. A large number of mothers attested to not perceiving malaria as a serious disease, as many of their children contracted mild cases of malaria. Hence, these mothers do not combat the disease at the first sign. A majority of these migrant mothers take a window period of two to three days to monitor the child. Also, professional medical attention, if sought for, mostly occurred when the health condition of the child becomes worse and out of control by the mothers.

Furthermore, the first instincts of the man is to act according to what they perceive to be of benefit to them. Results revealed that some international migrant mothers who are knowledgeable about malaria, and its causes, signs, and symptoms, including prevention and management strategies, seek professional help after administering first aid at home to their child. This is as a result of what they will benefit from in terms of quality of health-care services.

The basic orientation of the functionalism theory is premised on order and a functional society. Therefore, for a society to be so, it has to be void of any form of dysfunction. As a member of a society consisting of situations ranging from the family institution, educational institution, economic institution, religious institution, etc., every individual has a role to play to ensure the function, survival, and continuity of the society. The family is the smallest unit of the society, and it plays a very significant role in maintaining the stability, order, and survival of the society.

From research, results revealed that mothers as members of the society have very significant roles to play in the family institution. The health of the family relies basically on the shoulders of the mothers, who are nature's established caregivers while the fathers are saddled with the financial role, where they provide all funds to ensure that these mothers exercise their roles in caring for the family.

In summary, the health belief model in analysing the home management strategies of international migrant mothers with children under the age of five in the Akinyele local government area of Ibadan, Oyo state, centres on these mothers identifying their role in the society and engaging in proactive health behavior, based on how they perceive the condition, the severity, and the conditions necessary to promote health for their children and the family at large. This invariably results in long-term benefits for the society at large in terms of an improved standard of living condition and economic growth.

CONCLUSION

From this study, the research has been able to provide informed empirical and theoretical knowledge and findings on the sociological study of the home management of malaria amongst international migrant mothers in the Akin held local government area of Ibadan, Oyo state. This includes the level of knowledge of the international migrant mothers concerning the knowledge and practice of home management of malaria for their children under the age of five; how migrant mothers conduct and manage malaria for their children at home under the age of five; the perceived factors influencing respondents' choice of home management of malaria for their children under the age of five; the social relations involved in the practice of home management of malaria for their children under the age of five; the respondents' perception of home management of malaria; and the different ways to seek health care for children under the age of five. A theoretical discussion of findings was undertaken to further buttress the points on the dynamics involved in the home management of malaria by international migrant mothers with children under the age of five in the Akinyele local government area through the use of the health belief model.

Home management of malaria is a very important step in ensuring a controlled and sustainable health situation. This should be a first-aid management undertaken before proper diagnostics by profession health-care workers. The home management of malaria brings about the health benefits that are largely associated with health-seeking behaviors put in place that also ward off other diseases, such as cholera, typhoid, and many others. Therefore, environmental hygiene brings about environment protection and good health conditions for the Akinyele local government. Hence, improved health conditions also create economic benefits in return. As the saying goes, "Health is wealth." In the case of sound health for children, parents, especially the mothers, who are the primary care providers for the family, will not be limited in their economic pursuit and provide room for sustainable development. Children in return will fulfill their roles in society as well. However, issues such as unavailable financial resources, poor attitudes towards environmental hygiene, bad drainage systems, and poor housing construction are some of the challenges facing the home management of malaria by international migrant mothers with children under the age of five in the Akinyele local government area of Ibadan, Oyo state.

In all, the study was able to identify the importance of the home management of malaria at home and the roles played by actors at different levels: international migrant mothers, household members, friends, community health workers, and the government. In improving health standards and bringing about socioeconomic benefits to the people involved, the community, the state, and the nation at large, the government is successfully beginning to solve the problem of malaria in this population segment.

REFERENCES

Adebayo, A. M., Akinyemi, O. O., and Cadmus, E. O. 2015. 'Knowledge of Malaria Prevention among Pregnant Women and Female Caregivers of Under-five Children in Rural Southwest,' Nigeria. doi: 10.7717/peerj.792.

Adeboye, A. 2017. 'Fever: A Literature Review of Perceptions, Perspectives and Practices Traditional Medicine & Clinical Naturopathy Fever: A Literature Review of Perceptions, Perspectives and Practices,' (November). doi: 10.4172/2573-4555.1000249.

Birhanu, Z. et al. 2016. 'Malaria Related Perceptions, Care Seeking after Onset of Fever and Anti-Malarial Drug Use in Malaria Endemic Settings of Southwest Ethiopia,' *PLoS ONE*. doi: 10.1371/journal.pone.0160234.

Birhanu, Z., Yihdego, Y. Y., and Yewhalaw, D. 2017. 'Caretakers' Understanding of Malaria, Use of Insecticide Treated Net and Care Seeking-behavior for Febrile Illness of their Children in Ethiopia.' *BMC Infectious Diseases*, pp. 1–16. doi: 10.1186/s12879-017-2731-z.

Coleman, J. S. 1986. 'Social Theory, Social Research, and a Theory of Action,' *American Journal of Sociology*, 91(6), 1309–35. Available at: http://links.jstor.org/sici?sici=0002-9602%28198605%2991%3A6%3C1309%3ASTSRAA%3E2.0.CO%3B2-6.

Davis, R., Campbell. R, Hildon. R, Hobbs. Z. et al. 2015. 'Theories of Behaviour and Behaviour Change across the Social and Behavioural Sciences: A Scoping Review,' *Health Psychology Review*, 1–22. doi: 10.1080/17437199.2014.941722.

Edward, J. 2014. 'Undocumented Immigrants and Access to Health Care: Making a Case for Policy Reform,' *Policy, Politics, & Nursing Practice*. doi: 10.1177/1527154414532694.

Elsinga, J., Lizarazo, E F., Vincenti, M F., Schmidt, M., Velasco-, Z. I. 2015. 'Health Seeking Behaviour and Treatment Intentions of Dengue and Fever: A Household Survey of Children and Adults in Venezuela,' 1–18. doi: 10.1371/journal.pntd.0004237.

Goodwin, P. Y. and Garrett, D. A. 2005. 'Women and Family Health: The Role of Mothers in Promoting Family and Child Health,' *International Journal of Global Health and Health Disparities* 4(1), 30–42.

Hacker, K. Anies, M. F., Barbara L., Zallman, L. 2015. 'Barriers to Health Care for Undocumented Immigrants: a Literature Review,' *Risk Management and Healthcare Policy* 8, 175–83.

Journal, B. et al. 2014. 'Municipal Solid Waste Disposal And Environmental Issues In Kano Metropolis Nigeria.' Kaduna, Nigerian Defence Academy.

Kio, J. O., Agbede, C. O., Olayinka, F. E., Omeonu, P. E., Dire-arimoyo, Y. 2016. 'Knowledge, Attitudes and Practices of Mothers of Under-Five Regarding Prevention of Malaria in Children: Evidence from Ogun State, Nigeria.' doi: 10.9790/0837-2108080107.

Kwabe, T. S., Abdulfatai, O., Agbam, E. F., Usman, A., & Bashiru, A. M. (2013). Mothers Management of Malaria Fever among Under-Five Nomadic Fulani Children of Northeastern Nigeria. *American Journal of Infectious Diseases and Microbiology* 1(2), 26–33.

Ogula, O. D. 2015. *Research Methodology*. Rockstar, Washington DC: Hammesls Publications.

Olasunde, D. P. 2016. "Circular Migration Patterns and Determinants in Nairobi Slum Settlements." *Demographic Research* 23(20), 549–86.

Olugbade, O. T., Adedire, E., Ladipo, O. et al. 2014. 'Malaria Surveillance System Evaluation, Oyo State,' (June). doi: 10.1016/j.ijid.2014.03.992.

Parsons, T. (1951) *The Social System*. London, Tavistock Press.

Salami, K. K. and Umego, N. L. 2015. 'Household Environment and Malaria in Pregnancy in Ibadan, Nigeria,' *Health*, 10, 403–21. doi: 10.4236/health.2018.

Sangowawa, A. O. et al. 2014. 'Factors Associated with a Poor Treatment Outcome among Children Treated for Malaria in Ibadan, Southwest Nigeria,' *Epidemiology Research International*. doi: 10.1155/2014/974693.

Tarkang, E. E., and Zotor, F. B. 2015. 'Application of the Health Belief Model (HBM) in HIV Prevention: A Literature Review,' *Central African Journal of Public Health* 1(1), 1–8. doi: 10.11648/j.cajph.20150101.11.

World Health Organization. 2015. Annual Report on Malaria and Migration.

Ye, A., Win, N., Maung, T. M., Wai K. et al. 2017. 'Understanding Malaria Treatment—seeking Preferences within the Public Sector amongst Mobile/Migrant Workers in a Malaria Elimination Scenario: A Mixed—Methods Study,' *Malaria Journal*. BioMed Central, 1–13. Doi: 10.1186/s12936-017-2113-4.

United Nations. 2017. *2017 International Migration Report*. New York, UN Publications series.

Chapter 8

Malaria Control in Northern Nigeria

The Mosquito Eradication Campaign in Sokoto

Labbo Abdullahi

INTRODUCTION

The Sokoto province of northern Nigeria was a notorious mosquito hell-spot full of malarial germs. The traditional pattern of setting empty bottles on the tops of walls for security purposes, along with unsanitary conditions of the environment—pools, gutters, and drainages—provided breeding grounds for mosquito vectors in the area (Schram, 1971: 322). As such, throughout the colonial period, the most prevalent endemic ailment in Sokoto was malaria. Quite a number of colonial and missionary officials suffered from a serious malarial infection in the area (NAK/SOKPROF/FILENO/3120). The situation made Lugard consider the area unhealthy for habitation by expatriates, and almost every colonial and missionary official resented posting to the province because of malaria (GT Brit. Colonial Office/No.346). Until 1954, the British colonial officials and native authorities in the province employed several strategic campaigns to eradicate mosquitos and eventually malarial infection in the area. Public health regulations were enacted and enforced with regards to malaria control; there was weekly anti-mosquito work in the form of spraying of borrow-pits; there were intensive mosquito control campaigns in the Government Reservation Areas (GRAs); and routine spraying, oiling, draining, and filling measures were carried out in all stations (WJHCB/SOKPROF/1103). However, though mosquito vectors were restricted from the GRAs with the intensification of the idea of health-motivated residential segregation, the malarial infection continued unabated in the wider province up to 1954, when an all-inclusive campaign was embarked upon (AHAK/SNP/19/8/A.135). The 1954 mosquito-eradication campaign in Sokoto was a pilot scheme of the larger proposed malaria control project in northern Nigeria. The campaign was jointly sponsored by the Northern Regional Government, the Federal Malaria Service, the WHO, and UNICEF. The ultimate objective of the larger project was to eradicate mosquito vectors or control malaria transmission using sprayed insecticides in the rural areas of northern Nigeria, and the country at large (WJHCB/SOKPROF/2123). Although malaria transmission was not completely interrupted in the pilot area of Sokoto when the campaign ended in 1968, the scheme was said to be the most successful of such pilot campaigns in the country, and it tremendously reduced the incidence of malaria cases, especially among infants and children. This chapter examines the state of malarial infection and its control services before the choice of Sokoto for the pilot scheme, the roles of the major actors in the pilot scheme, and its upgrade to a full eradication campaign, as well as its transition to the WHO program of malaria prophylactic drug distribution in the area. Spraying activities are discussed, and the degrees of success recorded are assessed. In the final analysis, the chapter shows how best the scheme could be a lesson to the contemporary malaria eradication programs in the area and beyond.

BACKGROUND TO THE PREFERENCE OF SOKOTO AREA FOR THE PILOT PROJECT

The state of malarial infection and its persistence as a significant cause of morbidity in the Sokoto province attracted the choice of the area to pilot a mosquito-eradication campaign by the northern Nigerian government in 1954. Throughout the colonial period, the most prevalent ailments in the Sokoto province were malaria, bronchial troubles, and tropical ulcers. There were several outbreaks of epidemics, with some recorded deaths, such as from cerebral spinal meningitis, for instance, in 1906 (NAK/SOKPROF/FILENO.977), and smallpox in 1907 (NAK/SOKPROF/FILENO.39/1908). However, malaria was a common illness that attracted much of the attention of British colonial officials. This was perhaps because several British colonial officers were affected. For instance, in 1928, C.V. Scott and Mr. J.H. Smallwood, who were assistant divisional officers, suffered from serious cases of malaria that threatened their lives (NAK/SOKPROF/446/1928). Also, between 1936 and 1941, at least ninety-five but less than 120 total Europeans residing in the GRAs of Sokoto were reported to have suffered from malaria (AHAK/19/2/A.14). It is equally evident that the prevalence of malaria made some parts of the province uninhabitable to the missions. For instance, the closure of all the RCMs' stations in the Argungu Native Authority in 1948 was said to be due to prevalent malaria in the area (Connor, 2009: 59).

Given the malarial situation in the Sokoto province and coupled with the British experience of other diseases in their tropical colonies (Curtin, 1985: 594–613), British colonial officers in Sokoto prioritized anti-malaria measures, especially residential segregation (health-motivated residential segregation) (NAK/SOKPROF/FILENO.70/1919)[1] to distance themselves from the disease. They secluded themselves in the GRAs, and anti-malaria services, although carried out in the wider province, were prioritized in the government quarters (Labbo, 2018: 190). The services included weekly anti-mosquito work in the form of spraying of borrow-pits in some major towns of the province (WJHCB/SOKPROF/1103). The sprays in both the GRAs and the larger towns were under the supervision of a government mosquito control officer posted to the province. The mosquito-control services carried out in the GRAs and all other colonial officials' stations included routine spraying, oiling, draining, and filling. The services at the GRAs were funded by the government, while native authorities bore the financial responsibility of the few malaria-control services within their respective domains (AHAK/SNP/19/8/A.135).

Although mosquito vectors were finally restricted from the GRAs, inadequate funding and lack of regular supervision affected the exercise in towns; and thus, malaria continued to be the major cause of morbidity in the wider Sokoto province (AHAK/SNP/19/8/A.135). The level of malaria morbidity kept on increasing significantly. The government and the native authorities in the province continued to control malarial transmission with several programs in the GRAs and towns respectively. For instance, in 1951, a series of special mobile units were organized by the native authorities to carry out intensive anti-malaria services in towns (NAK/SOKPROF/FILENO.3601). However, malaria kept on recording about 40 percent of the total morbidity among the towns' populations (AHAK/SNP/19/2/A.21). As earlier mentioned, in the introduction, several reasons accounted for the persistent incidence of malaria in the Sokoto province. For instance, the traditional pattern of setting empty bottles on the tops of walls for security purposes (Schram, 322) and the ubiquity of pools, bad gutters, and unsanitary drainage became breeding grounds for mosquito vectors (WJHCB/SOKPROF/2123).

Consequent to the continued prevalence of malaria disease in the Sokoto province, several surveys were carried out to dig out the roots of the persistent malaria transmission in the area. There was, for example, a survey by a malariologist, Dr. H.M. Archibald, in September 1952, which concentrated on the Argungu Native Authority (a mosquito hell spot), where attendance figures for 1947–1950 obtained from the dispensary at Argungu showed that the number of cases diagnosed as malaria rose substantially during the three months of September to November following the rains. It was confirmed that breeding places of anopheles were widespread during the rainy season in pools, puddles, wells, and cattle hoofprints on the flooded marshy land (WJHCB/SOKPROF/2123). Similarly, Archibald, in collaboration with Mr. R.A. Fitz-John, mosquito control officer, and Mr. Roy Elliott, entomologist, undertook another survey in Sokoto and Gwandu Native Authorities during the wet season (July–August 1953). The survey revealed the prevalence of malaria in the area was an economic problem, and the disease caused appalling high infant mortality as well as diminished vitality, intelligence, and capacity to work amongst the adults. The disease was significantly prevalent during the critical farming season, when agricultural outputs and the general well-being of the population, whose margin between hunger and plenty was all too narrow, were affected (WJHCB/SOKPROF/2123).

With the persistence of malaria transmission as a great challenge to health care and the well-being of the people, the northern regional government decided to take the responsibility for malaria control in the rural areas of the region. The government initiated a mosquito-eradication project to control malaria transmission in rural areas. Consequent to the prevalence of mosquito vectors in the Sokoto province, as confirmed by the results of Archibald's surveys, Sokoto province, comprising Sokoto, Gwandu, and Argungu Native Authorities, were chosen for a pilot scheme of the project in 1954. Thus, a Mass Malaria Control Unit was established in Birnin-Kebbi, the headquarters of Gwandu Native Authority, as the centre of the scheme. The pilot scheme was a will-to-win campaign that persisted amidst various setbacks, which were surmounted by its staff through thick and thin to achieve the desired goals (NAK/SOKPROF/TOU/22).

THE ESTABLISHMENT OF A MASS MALARIA CONTROL UNIT IN BIRNIN-KEBBI IN 1954

It is said (Schram, 322–23; Labbo, 195; and AHAK/SOKPROF/SNP/19/23/A.3970) that the most interesting scheme for the promotion of public health in the 1950s and 1960s in Sokoto province was the mosquito-eradication campaign in the western part of the province. The objective of the pilot scheme was to carry out a relative scale pilot exercise of the project using sprayed insecticides in fairly densely populated rural areas of northern Nigeria, inhabited by 100,000 people. The Sokoto province was chosen because of its one wet season (July to September), and thus, hopes were pinned on an easier break in the transmission of malaria in the area (Schram, 320). Also, Sokoto might have been chosen for the pilot because it was a notorious mosquito hotspot area in northern Nigeria. Whichever the case may be, the pilot scheme intended to evaluate the results, not only in terms of reduced sickness, but also in the increased productivity of the population (WJHCB/SOKPROF/2123).

The scheme intended to control malaria transmission through the spray of residential areas with three insecticides: dieldrin, benzene hexachloride (BHC), and dichlorodiphenyltrichloroethane (DDT) (NAK/SOKPROF/TOU/22). The target of the spray was not the elimination of all mosquitoes and flies, but to kill the two species that transmitted malaria and also to reduce termites (WJHCB/SOKPROF/2123).[2] An area in Gwandu Native Authority with an estimated population of 100,000 was chosen as the best site for the first phase of the pilot. Eventually, the control area was expanded far beyond Gwandu Native Authority to include some parts of Argungu and Sokoto (WJHCB/SOKPROF/2123). At the commencement of the operation, control posts were established along all the roads to the sprayed area to prevent larger-scale importation of anopheles into the area. The posts were manned by spraying staff that sprayed all buses coming into the controlled area (WJHCB/SOKPROF/2123).

FINANCES AND SUPPLIES: THE ROLES OF THE STAKEHOLDERS

The pilot scheme, as earlier mentioned, was jointly sponsored by the Northern Regional Government, UNICEF, and WHO. UNICEF and WHO played a very vital role in the area of finances and supplies to the success of the scheme. For instance, UNICEF supplied the insecticides, Land Rovers, and other forms of transport, which were estimated at a rising cost of £9,527 in 1954/1955 to £22,391 in 1958/1959. The regional government, on the other hand, was responsible for the payment of salaries of the sprayers and other staff of the scheme. For example, it was estimated that the contribution of the regional government to the payment of salaries between 1954 and 1959 was £49,335 (Schram, 321–22). WHO and the Federal Malaria Service, on the other hand, contributed £6,300, and £3,700 within the first two years of the scheme respectively (WJHCB/SOKPROF/2123). All the needed vehicles for the scheme were made available by the UNICEF, and they bore the words "Grant from the United Nations Children's Fund, UNICEF to the Children of Nigeria, 1954" (*"Kyauta Daga Majalisar Dinkin Duniya,* UNICEF, *Zuwaga K'ananan Yaran Kasar Nijeriya,* 1954") (WJHCB/SOKPROF/2123).

Other stakeholders that played significant roles in the success of the scheme were the native authorities in the area. The Sokoto province was comprised of four native authorities, namely Sokoto, Gwandu, Argungu, and Yauri. The contributions of the native authorities were very substantial, both in cash and in kind. For example, on the commencement of the scheme in 1954, special sums of £4,680 and £650 were contributed by Gwandu and Argungu Native Authorities respectively (WJHCB/MED/2/II/SOKPROF). The two authorities further approved the payment of 2s per adult male tax-payer in addition to their normal tax in the sprayed areas to partially finance the cost of the scheme (AHAK/SOKPROF/SNP/19/2/A.14). Consequent to the introduction of the levy of 2s, the native authorities continued with their financial support to the scheme. In 1957/1958, the contributions of Sokoto and Argungu were £8,491 and £650 respectively. In addition, Argungu made a further contribution of £650 in 1959/1960. Similarly, the three years' contributions of the Gwandu Native Authority were £4,680 in 1957/1958, £5,805 in 1958/1959, and £4,323 in 1959/19560 (WJHCB/SOKPROF/MED/25). The reason Gwandu led the other native authorities in terms of contribution was that the larger part of Gwandu was within the scheme area. The Yauri Native Authority had never given any contribution because it was not part of the scheme (WJHCB/SOKPROF/25/7).

Also, the native authorities contributed significantly to the enforcement of public health regulations to ensure the success of the scheme. For the scheme, there came public health rules that authorised village and ward heads to direct occupiers of buildings to allow staff of the Mass Malaria Control Unit, particularly sprayers, to enter their compounds and premises in the course of their duties. The rules gave sprayers a permit for hitch-free entry of every compound in the sprayed area (NAK/SOKPROF/FILENO.5751D). Native authorities were very instrumental in the enforcement of the rules using their traditional security men (*Dogarai*), who rallied around alongside the spraying teams to ensure absolute compliance with the rules (Labbo, 194–95).

SPRAYING EXERCISE AND ASSESSMENTS TO 1960

The initial stage of the campaign began with mobile cinema shows by the Public Relations Office, Cinema Section. The cinemas toured around the whole target-controlled area showing a series of films dealing with issues on malaria control (WJHCB/SOKPROF/2123). Thereafter, the campaign commenced, and in its first phase, over eighty thousand buildings were sprayed with insecticides. The number of malaria-carrying mosquitoes had been greatly reduced, and an area of six hundred square miles was practically cleared of flies, bedbugs, and lice (AHAK/SOKPROF/SNP/19/2/A.13).

In order to assess the effectiveness of the spraying operations during the first stage, the mortality and morbidity of infants and young children were investigated. An annual detailed census was arranged in two villages, one within and the other outside the control area. Names and ages of all inhabitants were recorded, and each year a check of those who died was made to assess the mortality rate in each of the two villages. Similarly, a record of every pregnant woman was made, and the fate of the unborn baby was ascertained in the subsequent year (WJHCB/SOKPROF/2123). According to the census, the level of malaria reduced drastically in the sprayed area by 1955. Consequently, the target area of the pilot scheme was expanded tenfold into a mass campaign organized to control malaria in a population of one million people in 1956. The object of the expansion was to apply the knowledge gained from the first phase of the scheme to as wide an area as was feasible (WJHCB/SOKPROF/2123).

However, the results of the campaigns indicated that the satisfaction obtained in the measures against anopheles in 1954/1955 was not sustained in 1955/1956. This was because, in the area sprayed with dieldrin, A.gambiae reappeared (AHAK/SOKPROF/SNP/19/2/A.14).[3] The cause of the reappearance was investigated, and it was established that A.gambiae developed a strong resistance to dieldrin and to a lesser extent, BHC, but DDT proved irresistible. Therefore, it was decided to discontinue dieldrin, and instead, the campaign relied on BHC since DDT was not available. Despite the reemergence of A. gambiae in the dieldrin zone, substantial vector control was achieved throughout the sprayed areas. An incidental and potentially valuable observation was that termites had virtually disappeared from the buildings that were sprayed (AHAK/SOKPROF/19/23/A.395).

The expansion of the area under the pilot scheme in 1956 was made after an agreement was reached between the WHO and UNICEF to upgrade the pilot project into an eradication campaign. This was the period when the WHO changed its policy of malaria control to eradication of it throughout the whole world. The expanded programme was put into effect in April 1956. By the end of the year, it was estimated that 260,800 people benefited from the campaign, and about 174,800 huts were sprayed during the first cycle. The second cycle extended the coverage of the campaign to a population of 487,000 people. Fortunately, the health survey conducted after the two cycles of spraying with DDT showed a very substantial reduction in malaria transmission in children under the age of five (AHAK/SOKPROF/SNP/19/2/A.14).

Meanwhile, an assessment of the extended campaign was made using data on mortality and morbidity obtained from several maternity and children welfare clinics in the sprayed zone. Such clinics at Birnin-Kebbi and Argungu[4] towns were used to provide comparative data for the fact that the towns had some similarities and most importantly were both on the *Fadama* (riverine area). The former was within the spraying area while the latter was outside. The results of the assessment showed great improvement in malaria control in Birnin-Kebbi. Consequently, there was another extension of the control area in 1956/1957, and the third extension of the project was made in 1957/1958 (WJHCB/SOKPROF/2123).

During the 1956/1957 campaign, the sprayed area was divided into northern and southern circuits for spraying, as well as the circuits' spraying teams. Each team was headed by a superintendent (NAK/SOKPROF/TOU/22). Upon the completion of the campaign, all dwellings in the control area were sprayed twice with DDT (AHAK/SOKPROF/SNP/19/2/A.15). In the meantime, the campaign was followed by promising preliminary investigations. The transmission of malaria was almost eliminated in some areas of the Gwandu Native Authority using DDT. However, the transport problem became a major hitch to the project. The problem was mainly due to the poor state of the roads linking the villages. The problems caused slower work and increased difficulties for both staff and vehicles (AHAK/SOKPROF/SNP/19/2/A.15). Concerning the third extension in 1957/1958, a population of 435,582 people were sprayed; and since then, there was no further expansion of the control area (AHAK/SOKPROF/SNP/19/2/A.16).

On the whole, both the 1956/1957 and 1957/1958 campaigns were assessed through the examinations of sweeps at eight villages within the pilot projected area and at eight villages within the 1956/1957 and 1957/1958 extended areas. Special sweeps of the villages were arranged to see the limits of the interruption of transmission. The testimony to the success of the spraying was the fact that people no longer needed mosquito nets in the extended areas where DDT was used (NAK/SOKPROF/TOU/22). With regard to the achieved interruption of malaria transmission, the senior medical officer of the Zaria Medical Division, during his visit inspection, commented as follows: "Even in Birnin-Kebbi, previously a notorious mosquito hell-spot, I only noticed two culicines during my stay, and I saw none in Argungu" (NAK/SOKPROF/TOU/22).

However, the hopes to achieve complete interruption and eradication of malaria transmission were dashed because, as usual, during the rainy season of 1959, an appreciable number of vectors appeared in the sprayed area. Consequently, an investigation indicated that some villages had been unevenly sprayed with the DDT while others were adequately sprayed, but they still harboured vectors (Schram, 321–22). It was realized that the problem associated with the spraying campaign was that, despite the existing rules against noncompliance in the campaign, there was still a pocket of defiant people. For example, in 1959, about ten householders in the Yabo and Bodinga Districts of the Sokoto Native Authority refused to cooperate with the spraying teams. Most importantly, in the same year, the village head of the Sifawa Village Area of Sokoto, who was supposed to be instrumental in the hitch-free exercise, disallowed the sprayers' entry to his residence (WJHCB/SOKPROF/NA/MH/0013/S.1). But despite all the hitches, the campaign continued with its rigorous fight against malaria until 1960 (WJHCB/SOKPROF/NA/MH/0013/S.1).

POST-COLONIAL SPRAYS AND DISTRIBUTION OF MALARIA PROPHYLACTIC DRUGS TO 1972

By 1960, it was concluded that eradication of malaria could never be completely achieved. However, the campaign was popular and had reduced transmission to a fair level, hence, the regional government decided to continue with it after independence. Thus, the Mass Malaria Control Unit at Birnin-Kebbi continued to carry on with its responsibility of malaria control until it was scrapped in 1968 (Sokoto State Health Project, 1983: 28–30). The spraying and other control activities continued vigorously, and the general public became active and receptive to the services. For example, in 1961, eight hundred thousand huts were sprayed in the area of the scheme. Although the malaria transmission was not completely interrupted in the sprayed area, it was clear that infants and children in the controlled area were at an advantage compared to those in the unsprayed areas (AHAK/SOKPROF/SNP/19/2/A.19).

Meanwhile, UNICEF withdrew its assistance to the eradication campaign in 1962. But the regional government became fully responsible for the campaign (AHAK/SOKPROF/SNP/19/2/A.19). Thus, the level of control previously achieved was still maintained; with transmission reduced to a very low level and investigations on the behaviour of the mosquito vector, the diminishment of the relationship between parasite and the human host ensued (AHAK/SOKPROF/SNP/19/23/A.399). Similarly Sokoto, Gwandu, and Argungu Native Authorities continued to give financial assistance for the services; for instance, between 1960 and 1962, Gwandu contributed £4,500 to the campaign (WJHCB/SOKPROF/25/7).

WHO, on the other hand, continued to assist in the campaign and later institutionalized a new WHO Malaria Eradication Programme in the area. The new trend in the campaign came about when, in 1962, an agreement was signed by the WHO and the regional government for an eradication programme in northern Nigeria. In the agreement, the staff of the WHO was to cooperate with the government staff in a programme of research for the establishment of satisfactory eradication methods (AHA/SOKPROF/SNP/19//23/392).

Meanwhile, the usual spraying continued, and by 1962, a total of forty thousand square miles in some parts of Gwandu, Sokoto, and Argungu Native Authorities were sprayed (AHAK/SOKPROF/SNP/19/2/A.21). Spraying operations in the year included 384,654 huts sprayed within the first six months, and about the same number of huts were again sprayed in the subsequent six months (AHAK/SOKPROF/19/2/A.21).

WHO's Malaria Eradication Training School in Lagos embarked on a preliminary study of malaria services during the 1962 campaign as part of its pre-eradication project in the area. Through the study, technical data was collected, and a plan was prepared for institutionalizing a WHO Malaria Eradication Program in the Sokoto province based on the WHO-Northern Regional Government Agreement (AHA/SOKPROF/SNP/19//23/392). The study confirmed that malaria was common throughout the province, and there was no place in which it was not found. Severe and complicated attacks of malaria were seen more often in children than in adults. It was also ascertained that malaria killed, and a complicated attack of the disease must, therefore, be quickly and properly treated. Thus, malaria prophylactic drugs were recommended to be taken by everyone, especially children, in what was termed as a WHO Demonstration Zone (WJHCB/SOKPROF/MED/76). Hence, malaria services in the area ensued under the sponsorship of the regional government and the WHO until 1967, when a northwestern state was created. Thereupon, a State Malaria Control Board was constituted by the Executive Council of the State in 1968. The duties of the Board included advice on any matters connected with malaria control, initiation of investigation on any matter likely to promote control of malaria, and recommendations to the state government (WJHCB/SOKPRO/C/662/VOL.1).

However, it is pertinent to note that the support of the WHO was withdrawn in 1967, and while withdrawing, the WHO concluded that spraying exercises against mosquitoes at an enormous cost were not producing the expected results; therefore, it recommended an end to the exercise. Instead, the WHO advised the formation of an epidemiological unit; and consequently, the State Epidemiological Unit was established in 1969 (WJHCB/SOKPROF). With the emergence of the Unit, malaria control services continued, and from 1969, the services were mainly in the form of distributing anti-malaria drugs to all expectant mothers, children under the age of five, and all cases of fever within the control area. This scheme was prioritised between 1970 and 1972, when the state government ensured a regular and adequate supply of anti-malarial tablets to all the villages in the area (WJHCB/SOKPROF).

The distribution of anti-malaria drugs was limited to the WHO Demonstration Zone. The drug distributed was chloroquine syrup, administered orally to children assembled in villages (WJHCB/MED/28/VOL.I). During the process of drug administration, health educators were attached to the drug distribution team to publicise the scheme among the housewives and mothers of children. The essence was to convince them to bring their children for the receipt of the drugs and to make sure that the children swallowed the same. The expectant mothers were equally enlightened to take the drugs every fortnight. The work of prophylactic drug distribution went hand in hand with the treatment of several fever cases (WJHCB/MED/32/VOL.II). Although malaria transmission was not completely interrupted through spraying and the administration of anti-malarial drugs, there was a very remarkable achievement in which the incidence of malaria cases was greatly reduced in the control area, as indicated in the following tables showing the five-year mortality rate of malaria within and outside anti-malaria drug distribution zones respectively:

According to the comparative tables above, there is an indication of improvement in terms of malaria control within the Drug Distribution Zone, more so than outside the zone. For instance, there were 582 deaths caused by malaria in a population of 38,882 people within the non-control area, as compared to only 704 deaths in a higher population of 101,249 within the control area. Similarly, the infant mortality in the control area was 71 within total births of 2,700, while that in the non-control area was 96 within 1,237 total births. It is therefore clear that, though not up to the satisfactory level, success had been recorded. Unfortunately, from 1972, the work of malaria control in terms of spraying and drug administration began to be neglected. Consequently, malaria remained the most prevalent communicable disease in the area. For example, in 1980, malaria was recorded as 77 percent of the cases of communicable diseases (Sokoto State Health Statistics of 1980, 1982: 4–5). In 1981, malaria cases constituted 69 percent of all cases of communicable diseases (Sokoto State Health Statistics of 1981, 1981: 4). And in 1982, the cases of malaria disease had reached 64 percent of all communicable disease cases (Sokoto State Health Statistics of 1982, 1984: 3–4).

Table 8.1. Mortality in Anti-Malaria Drug Distribution Zone

Year	*Population*	*No. of Births*	*Infant Mortality*		*Child Mortality*		*Total Mortality*
1968	20,308	507	7	13%	26	8%	106
1969	20,679	543	16	29%	41	13%	169
1970	19,657	733	13	17%	13	4%	114
1971	20,197	468	17	36%	49	16%	158
1972	20,408	449	18	40%	25	8%	157
Total	**101,249**	**2,700**	**71**		**154**		**704**

Source: WJHCB/MED/28/VOL. I/Vaccination, 1967–1976

Table 8.2. Mortality Outside Anti-Malaria Drug Distribution Zone

Year	Population	No. of Births	Infant Mortality		Child Mortality		Total Mortality
1968	8,217	253	9	35%	23	19%	118
1969	8,201	237	17	71%	22	19%	126
1970	6,564	443	10	22%	29	22%	115
1971	8,024	325	17	52%	43	37%	128
1972	7,876	216	16	73%	24	20%	95
Total	**38,882**	**1,237**	**69**		**141**		**582**

Source: WJHCB/MED/28/VOL. I/Vaccination, 1967–1976

CONCLUSION

The chapter discussed the campaign that started as a pilot scheme and developed into a full mosquito eradication project, eventually ending as a malaria-control programme by the use of prophylactic drugs. Also, examined in the discourse, the campaign included the roles of such stakeholders as the northern regional government, the Federal Malaria Control, UNICEF, the WHO, and the native authorities in the province. From the discourse, it is clear that all the concerned actors made the best of their efforts to control the incidence of malaria and its resultant mortality in the province through mosquito eradication and the distribution of prophylactic drugs. With regards to the spraying of insecticides against mosquito vectors, a lot of funds were expended. For instance, the total cost of the activities was approximated at about £65,000 per annum, and for that amount, almost half a million people benefited twice each year (AHAK/SOKPROF/SNP/19/23/A.398). Although the vectors and malaria infections kept on reemerging, the stakeholders and the malaria control staff, especially sprayers, put in their very best and minimized the rates of malarial morbidity and mortality. Consequently, the project was rated as the first of its kind in terms of coverage and success in the whole of British West Africa (AHAK/SOKPROF/SNP/19/23/A.397 and Schram, 322).

Regarding the lesson for contemporary anti-malaria services, the discourse in the chapter revealed that not just the persistence of malaria with the highest morbidity and mortality in the contemporary Sokoto area and beyond is linked to the lack of vector control and poor sanitation, but the disease is preventable with the use of mosquito-killing insecticides and malarial prophylactic drugs as done in the past. This is because it is clear that stagnant water in poorly drained areas where mosquitoes multiplied and spread every minute continued to be common everywhere in Sokoto and other northern Nigerian malaria-endemic areas; and as such, malarial infections persisted. Therefore, the need to resuscitate the already-existing programmes and reintroduce new programmes and activities of environmental sanitation, spraying of insecticides against mosquito vectors, and large-scale distribution of malaria-prophylactic drugs is imperative in the contemporary anti-malaria campaign in Nigeria.

REFERENCES

AHAK/19/2/A.14/Provincial Annual Report for 1956.

AHAK/SNP/19/2/A.21/Provincial Annual Report for 1963.

AHAK/SNP/19/8/A.135/Nigerian Annual Report on the Medical Services for the Year 1953/1954.

AHAK/SOKPROF/19/2/A.21/Provincial Annual Report for 1963.

AHAK/SOKPROF/19/23/A.395/Annual Report of the Ministry of Health Northern Nigeria for the Year 1955/1956.

AHAK/SOKPROF/SNP/19/2/A.13/Provincial Annual Report for 1955.

AHAK/SOKPROF/SNP/19/2/A.14/Provincial Annual Report for 1956.

AHAK/SOKPROF/SNP/19/2/A.15/Provincial Annual Report for 1957.

AHAK/SOKPROF/SNP/19/2/A.16/Provincial Annual Report for 1958.

AHAK/SOKPROF/SNP/19/2/A.19/Provincial Annual Report for 1961.

AHAK/SOKPROF/SNP/19/2/A.21/Provincial Annual Report for 1962.

AHAK/SOKPROF/SNP/19/23/A.397/Annual Report of the Ministry of Health Northern Nigeria for the Year 1960.

AHAK/SOKPROF/SNP/19/23/A.398/Annual Report of the Ministry of Health Northern Nigeria, 1961.

Connor. E.O. 2009. *From the Niger to the Sahara: The Story of the Archdiocese of Kaduna.* Ibadan: Intec Printers.

Curtin. P.D. 1985. "Medical Knowledge and Urban Planning in Tropical Africa." *American Historical Review*, 90(3).

GT Brit. Colonial Office/No.346/Colonial Reports-Annual/Northern Nigeria/Report for the period from 1st Jan, 1900 to 31st Mar, 1901.

Hightingale. C.H. 2012. *Segregation: A Global History of Divided Cities.* Chicago and London: University of Chicago Press.

Labbo. A. 2018. "A History of Modern Medical and Healthcare Services in Colonial and Post-Colonial Sokoto Province, 1920–1986. Department of History, Usmanu Danfodiyo University, Sokoto: *PhD Thesis*.

NAK/SOKPROF/446/1928/Sokoto Provincial Annual Report for 1928.

NAK/SOKPROF/FILENO.3120 and NAK/SOKPROF/FILENO.446/1928.

NAK/SOKPROF/FILENO.3601/Medical Policy.

NAK/SOKPROF/FILENO.39/1908.

NAK/SOKPROF/FILENO.5751D.

NAK/SOKPROF/FILENO.70/1919.

NAK/SOKPROF/FILENO.977/1906.

Schram. R. 1971. *A History of the Nigerian Health Services.* Ibadan: Ibadan University Press.
Sokoto State Health Project. Feasibility Report. February 1983. MOCO Nigeria Limited. Lagos Nigeria, Chap. 2.
Sokoto State Health Statistics of 1980. January: 1982. Statistic Division. Ministry of Economic Planning. Sokoto. Nigeria.
Sokoto State Health Statistics of 1981. 1981. Statistic Division. Economic Planning Department. Ministry of Finance and Economic Planning. Sokoto State. Sokoto.
Sokoto State Health Statistics of 1982. January: 1984. Statistic Division. Ministry of Economic Planning. Sokoto. Nigeria.
WJHCB/MED/2/II/SOKPROF/Development of NA Dispensary and Hospitals in Sokoto.
WJHCB/MED/28/VOL.I/Vaccination, 1967–1976.
WJHCB/MED/32/VOL.II/Malaria Control Project, 1970–1973.
WJHCB/SOKPRO/C/662/VOL.1/State Malaria Control Board 1968–1968.
WJHCB/SOKPROF/1103/Kebbi Town European Reservation and Sanitation of Mosquito Control.
WJHCB/SOKPROF/1103/Kebbi Town European Reservation and Sanitation of Mosquito Control.
WJHCB/SOKPROF/2123/Pilot Malaria Control Project.
WJHCB/SOKPROF/25/7/Malaria Control Campaign Expenditure from Special Levy Account.
WJHCB/SOKPROF/Malaria Control Scheme in Western Sokoto.
WJHCB/SOKPROF/MED/25/Malaria Pilot Control Scheme Policy 1955–1971.
WJHCB/SOKPROF/MED/76/Anti-malaria Drugs 1964–1966.
WJHCB/SOKPROF/NA/MH/0013/S.1/Malaria Control Survey and Treatment: Correspondence.

NOTES

1. The idea of health-motivated residential segregation began when Joseph Chamberlain, the colonial secretary, ordered all West African governors to scout areas that could be reserved for European residence. Consequently, "Colonial Office's Disease Theory of Segregation" was enforced. In northern Nigeria, Lugard embarked on residential segregation schemes in line with the theory. He formulated an ordinance that segregated some areas called "GRAs" for Europeans. GRAs were separated by a 440-yard-wide "Building Free Zone" with a view to keeping Europeans away from diseases, especially malaria. In his first Annual Report of Northern Nigeria (1900), Lugard says: "I have it in contemplation to gradually move the native town six or seven miles downstream, and so to do away with the pollution of the water, and with other evils such as . . . the infection of mosquitoes with malarial germs. . . . Moreover, the British continued to distance themselves from malarial infection through health motivated segregation policy. For example, there was an Ordinance in 1917, which imposed fines on Europeans, including businessmen who lived outside their

reservation. In 1919, there was a total isolation of the British officers from the people of the Sokoto Province in which the latter, were prohibited to go to the Government Reserve Areas" (GT Brit. Colonial Office/No.346 and Hightingale, 2012: 176–80).

2. The insect-killing chemical was sprayed in water onto all walls and ceilings; when the water dried, a layer of powder was left on the surfaces, and it was the powder that killed the insects. The powder remained powerful for six months after spraying. It poisoned those mosquitoes that rested on it so that it was not effective when covered by a fresh surface of mud plaster and or it got brushed off the walls. The chemicals were not poisonous to larger creatures, so there was no fear of harming domestic animals or poultry. Humans were quite safe, but as an added precaution, measures were taken to ensure that the spray was not allowed to fall onto food. The sprayers tried to put a layer of powder onto every surface on which a mosquito might rest inside a building. The chemicals used did not, however, kill immediately; therefore, mosquitoes were seen resting on a treated wall and later flew off apparently unharmed. They more often than not had already picked up enough poison to kill them soon after. The rationale behind the gradual method of killing insects was to avoid discouraging them from coming into a house because the major aim was to attract and kill them. The major hope was that mosquitoes were to be poisoned before they had time to lay their eggs, and that their ability to reproduce was thus interrupted.

3. Originally, for the experimental purpose, the mapped area for the scheme was divided into three sectors, and each sector was sprayed with a different drug: dieldren, BHC, and DDT. Observation since then indicated that some mosquitoes were developing a resistance to spraying. Late in 1955, proof was obtained of the resistance to dieldren by *Anopheles Gambiae*, one of the main vectors. Further research both in London and in the field by WHO staff proved that this mosquito was resistant to BHC also, but not DDT, and this discovery had excited international interest. It had also caused a change in the spraying plan, where DDT had to replace as soon as adequate supplies are available both BHC and dieldren.

4. It is pertinent to clarify that although the Argungu Native Authority was in the target sprayed area, not all the towns and villages of the native authority were under the sprayed zone, including the Argungu town itself. But Birnin-Kebbi town of Gwandu Native Authority, on the other hand, was one of the towns included in the sprayed area.

Chapter 9

Maternal Health Experiences of Women in the Farm Settlement Areas of the Akwa Ibom State

Moses Idongesit Peters, Nsidibe A. Usoro, and Aniekan Etim Bassey

INTRODUCTION

One of the common health effects in marginal communities is maternal and health care services (MCHS). Maternal health has been a great important factor in the pursuit of the health sector and health development in third-world countries, especially within the rural regions of sub-Saharan Africa, where it remains a great battle among stakeholders in the health sector. The fight against death among women of reproductive age and children between birth and five years of age has been a fight to sustain humanity and human reproduction in sub-Saharan Africa. As important as the subject matter is in comparison to the various undertaken actions by various stakeholders, the case is still reported to be a continuous challenge, as new causes of morbidity and mortality related to MCHS are discovered every year. The newly emergent dimensions and cases demand critical sectorial analysis and intervention approaches for effective solutions. Despite the progress attained by the stakeholders in the fight against maternal and infant mortality, as of 2020, forty-seven children under the age of one died for every one thousand live births (Statista, 2022). Developed nations like the United States and Germany have recorded a one-in-4,700 death rate resulting from complications in pregnancy, as compared to one in thirty-nine in Africa (UNFPA, 2013), making these health cases a serious situation within the continent. Maternal health still remains a great combating issue within every health post, health centre, and hospital found within the continent of Africa.

Maternal health is generally said to refer to health-care services provided for women throughout pregnancy, during childbirth, and in the postnatal period, and each of these stages should be a positive experience in order to ensure the safety of the mother's life and her baby (WHO, 2022). Maternal health reveals the health needs of a woman of reproductive age, which is mostly agreed to be between fifteen to forty-nine years of age. These health needs are mostly increasing in the low-income countries (LMCs) among the developing countries of the world. The concerns of women and children's health have caused an expansion in the subject matter that has led to the reproductive, maternal, newborn, and child health (RMNCH) concept that merges the health issues and its interventions throughout the life spans of women before and during pregnancy, and newborn babies from their first day to their fifth birthday (World Bank, 2016). UNFPA (2013) reported that 287,000 women died from complications resulting from pregnancy, twenty to thirty women suffered from severe anaemia, damage to the reproductive organs, severe postpartum disability (such as obstetric fistula), and chronic pain or infertility, despite the fact that about half of the 123 million women received antenatal, delivery, and newborn care every year (UNFPA, 2013).

Maternal and infant mortality are preventable health challenges. The WHO (2019) reports that developed nations like Norway, Sweden, and Australia, among others, have put more resources toward curbing the health challenges of their nations as compared to the developing nations. UNICEF (2009) stated that many women in developing nations give birth at home without skilled or professional health-care workers present, yet their newborns are usually healthy and survive past their first few weeks of life, even throughout their fifth birthday, and despite the multitude of risks associated with pregnancy and childbirth, some of mothers also survived, while some lost their lives. According to Lassi, Salam, Das, and Bhutta (2014), poor maternal, newborn, and child health-care services have over the decades remained a visible health challenge among the low- and middle-income countries(L&MICs), especially in sub-Saharan Africa. According to UNICEF (2009), creating an enabling environment for safe motherhood and childbirth directly depends on the capacity to make available care and attention for pregnant women and their newborns by communities and families, the ability of skilled health workers, and the availability of adequate health-care facilities, equipment, and medicines and emergency care when needed.

Having a newborn baby is culturally a thing of joy among legally married couples, and it is a joyful experience to hold a safely delivered baby, even those born to mothers who were impregnated illegally in one way or the other. The road to delivery, the delivery experience, and the duties of caring for the infants have cost the lives of many mothers and innocent babies, and children under the age of five years still suffer morbidity and mortality in many developing nations of the world. WHO (2019) reports that most maternal mortality occurs in the developing countries, which has caused disparities in the health statistics between the developed nations and the developing nations. Apart from death, many mothers have survived these experiences, but they are left behind with difficult illnesses to hold to drugs and other medical attentions as they live. The challenge of putting in place safety measures for proper medical attention for pregnant women, mothers, and infants has been facing the people, communities, and governments in the world, and it is most demanding in third-world countries. UNFPA (2013) further reports that there are very few properly equipped health facilities in developing countries to take care of the maternal health care of women, and those that do exist are rarely capable of meeting the needs of women and their babies.

Nigeria has been facing great challenges in the quest to attain development due to the inability of the government to meet the health needs of the populace over the decades since her independence. Despite the decline in maternal mortality in some parts of the world, Nigeria has been battling with the challenge of meeting the needs of reproductive women in many areas and regions of the nation, especially with the struggle against child marriage and traditionally accepted polygamy among many ethnic groups of the nation. According to Izugbara, Wekesah, and Adedini (2016), despite the global decline in maternal mortality since the 1990s, the maternal health experience continues to be risky for millions of Nigerian women who have seen death and disability in many regions, states, and communities in Nigeria. Izugbara, Wekesah, and Adedini (2016) further report that the maternal health care system in Nigeria is in such a pathetic state involving orthodox, faith-based, and traditional health providers who are local injectionists, itinerant medicine hawkers, and patent medicine sellers. These quacks or fake medical providers have jeopardized the lives of innocent women and children through filling the gaps widened by the lack of formal health-care service providers by selling merchandise in buses, markets, streets, and motor parks. While spiritualists, through incantations and prayers, are taking their own share through the laying on of hands, the ingestion of materials, and the use of holy water and oil (Izugbara, Wekesah, & Adedini, 2016).

The Anderson health-care utilization model was adopted for a theoretical framework of the study. According to Okumagba (2011), Anderson, and Neuman (1975), grouped in three sequences, a cluster of factors, which are predisposing, enabling, and need factors are capable of influencing health-care utilization behavior. Anderson's model on health-care services utilization explains the key health challenges and experiences of the study participants, which include the identification of the need for maternal health care services. The predisposing factor is the pregnant women and their infants, which are accompanied by health complications among women of reproductive age in the farm settlement areas. Their farm produces generated income, which is the enabling factor for the utilization of maternal health-care services if available, and an absence of maternal health-care services providers and health-care facilities in the farm settlement areas affects their ability to access and utilize maternal health-care services and cope with daily maternal health challenges. The vulnerability of mothers and their children to health complications and illnesses creates the need for maternal health-care services and the provision of health-care facilities for farm settlement areas/ communities.

The study was carried out in a marginalized farm settlement community. The Isohidim farm settlement area, by geographical location, is a large farm community surrounded by water, which makes entrance to the community difficult, due to wooden bridges set over the rivers by the farmers. The surrounding water makes the environment a haven to mosquitos. Since people are always scared of the durability of wooden bridges, the community seems to have been abandoned by the government of the day and other organizations who are supposed to reach out to the people living within the farm settlement community. Though they are farmers, and their products include cassava, maize, okra, pepper, turmeric, ginger, and other food crops like potatoes, some of the people go hunting for bush-meat production and tapping for palm-wine production, together with farming.

The lack of accessibility to this farm settlement community affects their economy due to the lack of proper roads and transportation systems, thereby allowing those who come into the community to exploit them of their produce by buying in low prices with the basis of bearing the cost of transporting the produce to the towns and cities for markets. The farm settlement community is marginalized in terms of health care. This is because they do not have any health-care facilities in the community or near the community, nor do the health workers especially during community immunization easily go into the farm settlement communities unless the community leaders make special arrangements for them.

This research report is part of an ethnographic study carried out in farm settlement areas in Akwa Ibom State. Qualitative research techniques were adopted to obtain information on the maternal health experiences of women of reproductive age among farmers in Isohidim farm settlement area in the Ibeno local government area, Akwa Ibom State. In-depth interviews, key informants (KII), and participant observation were utilized. Most of the participants were interviewed using interview schedules at their farmlands, and some were in the convenience of their homes.

The study participants consist of a convenience sample of farmers in the Isohidim farm settlement area in the Ibeno local government area, in Akwa Ibom State, who merely expressed their consent to participate in the study. The researchers adopted a big-net approach (Fetterman, 2010) to capture the sample size, which was drawn from all interviewed participants through a snowballing technique. In-depth interviews and participant observation were used for data collection. The interviews were concerning issues relating to the maternal health experiences of women of reproductive age in the farm settlement area in Akwa Ibom State.

Data were collected to examine the level of availability of maternal health-care services, the level of accessibility of maternal health care by women of reproductive age, and alternative measures engaged by women in the farm settlement area to meet their maternal and reproductive health needs. These examined variables generated data for the maternal health-care experiences of women in the settlement. Though the interview schedule for the study was developed in the English language, interviews with the participants were conducted in both the English and Ibibio languages.

The farm settlement areas in Akwa Ibom State have suffered much neglect by the state government in the area of providing social amenities to citizens within these rural areas, which makes them marginalized communities in the state. The absence of government intervention in the farm settlements has made life very difficult for the farmers, with women and children being at the worst receiving ends. Health care is of great importance to the survival of the farmers living within the settlement areas. Therefore, the absence of formal health-care services is the absence of formal maternal and reproductive health-care services for women of reproductive age and their infants. In the available literature on maternal health care, much has been said on the issues as they affect different women in different areas and communities, but the maternal and reproductive health-care of women in farm settlements has not been given the needed attention, which is the gap this research work sought to fill. Against this backdrop, this research examined the maternal health-care experiences of women of reproductive age in the Isohidim farm settlement area in the Ibeno local government area of Akwa Ibom State.

FINDINGS

Availability of Maternal Health-Care Services

Emerging from observations and discussions about the availability of health-care facilities for the provision of maternal health-care services were the helpless situations always encountered by the farmers whenever health-care needs arise, and the vulnerability of pregnant women and their infants to health crises due to the absence of a formal health-care facility in the farm settlement area. One of the community elders in the Isohidim farm settlement area explained that they do not have any hospital, health-care centre, medicine store, or pharmacy to provide for the maternal health-care needs of their wives and daughters in the settlement area or in any neighbouring farm settlement community within their reach. One of the study participants, in her narrative, reported that:

> Me and my husband started to live here over twenty years ago, and since we came here, up till now, we have never had any health centre, any hospital, or any private person come here for hospital business. So, we are really suffering, especially we women during pregnancy and delivery, and even the babies and children are suffering. We do not have even a chemist to buy drugs from here because all of us here are farmers and the only person that came for chemist business parked out to Mkpanak after he got married to his wife, because his wife did not want to live with him here in the farm community. The government is not even trying at all. They will come here and talk to us during election time, and we will vote with Akpansung. All the farm communities, we will vote together. But after that, they will go, and we will not see them again. Our husbands talked to them about roads, hospital, schools, and electricity. They will promise and swear by thunder that they will make sure we have them. Immediately after election, *piam, piam, piam*, they pack up and go and leave us us the way you people see us now. No hospital, nothing. (Eka, 45 years, farmer/ women group leader)

Among the visible characteristics of the Isohidim farm settlement area includes the absence of a health-care facility, the absence of any health-care services provider, the absence of any medicine store or pharmacy, and the absence of any health workers, making accessibility to maternal health-care services a great challenge. The availability of maternal health-care services remains a serious challenge among the farmers in the Isohidim farm settlement area. Though there exist the knowledge of availability of maternal health-care services in health-care centres and hospitals outside the farm settlement area, having it closer to them and within their reach remains an expectation that, according to the study participants, they believe will one day happen through the health-care intervention programmes of either the government, non-governmental agencies, or some private individual. The expectation of availability and accessibility of maternal health-care services by many of the farmers in the farm settlement communities is a great hope.

Gathered information through interviews reveals the bitter experiences the farmers have undergone due to the absence of maternal and reproductive health-care services providers. Narratives from study participants outlined the losses and the pain-bearing lifestyles of the farmers. Some of the women who were part of the study lamented on the lives of women and children who have been lost in the farm settlement area, especially during child delivery, due to the absence of maternal health-care service providers and medical professionals or health workers in the Isohidim farm settlement community. One of the study participants in her narratives said:

> We have suffered a lot living here, and most times we feel we have invested our lives in these communities and we cannot just leave like that. This is our village, though we have lost women and children to death because we hardly have access to maternal health-care services from any doctor, nurse, or even a pharmacist. None of these people want to come and do business here because there are no social amenities here. We have lost our children to death, and we wept and moved on. Go around and see it for yourself. (Slimmy, 43, farmer/charcoal trader)

Another participant in her narratives reported that:

> The government has abandoned us to our fate. But we have been voting during the elections. They have refused to help us. Our women used to die at the entrance bridge, which you saw while coming into this community, and their unborn children died with them, because some of them couldn't have the boldness to walk through the woods in labour, and out of fear, they chose to cry, wept, and suffered in pain. Some of them did give birth by the bridge due to fear of crossing the bridge, especially in the night. Some of them who couldn't give birth at the bridge, died at the bridge. We couldn't save them because we do not have any professional maternal health-care service providers here; we do not have Western medicines or somebody to prescribe them. Even if we do have someone to prescribe them, we will still have to go to Ukpenikang, Mkpanak, or Eket to buy such prescribed drugs or call for professional services. (Affi, 63, farmer)

In the case of availability of maternal health-care services for the farmers in the Isohidim farm settlement area in the Ibeno local government area, as gathered from interviews, it was gathered that there are no maternal health-care services at Isohidim. This is due to the absence of health-care facilities that are supposed to provide such services to the farmers within the settlement area. Narratives revealed that the farmers and their families have suffered a lot and lost many women and children due to the absence and lack of medical facilities and maternal health-care services. Their health challenges and living in the absence of what is known to be available elsewhere has forcefully placed the people in pain of their expectations and the hope of having maternal health-care services available in the farm settlement areas of Akwa Ibom State.

Accessibility of Maternal Health-Care Services

Gathered information through interviews, discussions, and observation about the levels of the accessibility of maternal health-care services showed that most people in the Isohidim community do not have access to maternal and reproductive health care because of the absence of medical facilities in the farm settlement area under study. The few families who decided to utilize such care services have had to travel to other communities and neighbouring local government areas to get access to maternal health-care services. The community elders in their narratives reported that their women and children hardly have access to maternal health care since there is no available health-care facility in the farm settlement. One of the Isohidim community elders stated:

> We are tired of having to travel to get those medical services from neighboring communities. Since the government does not care enough about us to give the farm settlement communities at least one health-care centre, we do not worry over such again because we have suffered many things and nothing will scare us again. So, what I am telling you is that we do not have access to medical services, and we do not use those foreign drugs here. (Steve, 60, palm wine tapper)

Farmers from the Isohidim settlement area lamented the high cost of transportation—up to one thousand naira to Eket and Ukpenikang, which are about 60 kilometres and 40 kilometres respectively—in other to have access to maternal health care, and the cost of the medicine, which over time places serious financial and time concerns on the farmers. Discussions on whether they can get access to maternal health care and where they get it from due to the absence of medical or health-care facilities revealed that most of the women in Isohidim do not bother with accessing maternal health care during the initial stages of their pregnancy. Some of the women will have to endure health issues accompanying their pregnancies until they reach their last trimester or the last week before their expected delivery date (EDD). Often they begin to observe signs of labour before they will go out of the farm settlement to a hospital located in either Ukpenikang or Eket. One of the study participants, during her discussion and interview, reported that:

> We have been suffering here, especially we women and our children. Hmm, you will not believe that we have buried many children here in these farmlands that sometimes we are forced and tempted to believe that their spirits have blessed our farmlands because they understand and see our sufferings for them without any help. Most times, we have to wait when we are pregnant and endure whatever happens until it is near the delivery time. We often begin to see signs of labor before we can pack our things and go out to stay in the hospital and wait

> for delivery. Sometimes some of us stay for over a month because maybe we began to feel sick or had pains before the delivery month; this makes the hospital bills very expensive for something that we could have been going from our houses to the clinic if we had one in any of the farm settlement areas, even at Akpansung, which is a close farm settlement to us. But nobody cares about us apart from coming to buy foodstuffs and get us to vote in the elections. (Esty, 42, farmer/trader)

Emerging from interviews, discussions, and observations on why the farmers do not access maternal health care is the discovery that the absence of health facilities, financial burdens, and geographical distance to available health facilities outside the farm settlement areas are factors hindering or impeding the accessibility of maternal health-care services by women of reproductive age in the Isohidim farm settlement area. Most of the study participants agreed that the most important reason they do not have access to maternal health-care services remains the non-availability of a health-care facility in the farm settlement area. These have kept the farmers from accessing maternal and reproductive health-care services against their desire despite the pathetic health challenges faced by women of reproductive age in the Isohidim farm settlement area. One of the study participants narrated that:

> Our women do not have access to that kind of care and services. The hospital or health clinic that is supposed to give them such medical care is not found here, we don't have one, and the nurses who are supposed to render such services to our women are not here. You cannot find any here because the people who are supposed to know that we are Ibeno people and we are in need of medical care, too, our women and children, do not care about us in any way. We usually have to send our wives to our friends, relatives, and some customers for them to stay with them for a while, and in some cases, after delivery, until the baby is like three months. Then we go and pick them up. We do that so they can stay where they can easily have access to proper medical care. But it is not everybody here who has such connections. (Fri, 58, farmer/trader)

The discovery from the narratives concerning the level of accessibility of maternal health care among farmers in farm settlement areas under the study shows that farmers in the Isohidim farm settlement do not have access to maternal health-care services based on many reasons, of which the most important is the absence of a medical health-care facility within the farm settlement areas. This important reason has caused the deaths of many women and children, and created unmet health challenges of women, children, and even mature men within the farm settlement areas.

Alternatives Measures Engaged by Farmers for Maternal Health-Care Services

Information gathered through in-depth interviews, discussions, and observations concerning alternative measures engaged by women of reproductive age in the Isohidim farm settlement area revealed that the farmers have, over the years, developed a dependency on elderly women, who have, over the years, had experiences in child delivery in the settlement areas in providing maternal and reproductive care. The women have also found a dependency on the use of local herbs and faith healing for their health needs, due to the absence of medical health-care facilities to meet their maternal, reproductive, and other health needs. This dependency has generated bitter experiences for women and children, with a direct impact on families within the farm settlement areas. Collected data reveals that their dependency on elderly women for their maternal health care—who act as traditional birth attendants (TBAS)—and on local herbs has become strong over the years, and it has become part of their health belief systems. These elderly women, according to findings, have started leaving the area for training in order to gain more knowledge on birth attendance. Because they are agriculturists and due to the nature of their occupation, belief in the efficacy of local herbs seems to be a common cultural practice, which makes it easy to limit the effects of the absence of modern medical facilities in the farm settlements. One of the participants in her narrative reported that:

> We are no longer worried in some cases as we used to be worried, though in some difficult cases, some of us do suffer. But we have been praying, and God has reduced the number of difficult cases among us, such that we now rarely have such cases as we used to have before, especially as we now have some women, like traditional birth attendants (TBAs), who have started taking care of some pregnancy cases from the early stages. This is unlike before, when they were not going for training, but were only trying based on their experiences to assist younger women who could not go out of the farm areas for delivery on time or those who couldn't cross the bridge because of fear. Then we used to suffer many deaths. But now they are trying, because they go for training, and we contribute transport money for them to go for the training at Ukpenikang. (Ima, 38, farmer/hairstylist)

Dependency on alternative measures for maternal health care by women of reproductive age in Isohidim is built on the absence of health-care facilities and health workers within the farm settlement areas. Looking for the alternatives, according to the study participants, became imperative, since they couldn't wait and watch their children die and the women suffer, while some of their women died too. Narratives revealed that the elders of the communities had to look for a solution within their reach. While they trusted the lives of their young women to the elderly women in their maternal health, engaging in local herbs, others relied on church faith–based healing within the farm settlement area. A study participant during an interview narrated that:

> It is a long time since we decided to see how to fight back so we can see how to rescue our wives and children from dying every year on the farm. So, we decided to trust older women, our mothers, to help our wives and infants from dying like fowl every year, and we try roots and herbs because we have them enough here. What we have today is a bit better than what used to happen here. Maybe before, as you people were coming into this place, you would have seen us mourning or trying to bury a woman, or maybe a young child. My brethren, we have seen a lot here, but thanks be to God, who has not left us completely. (Eti, 43, hunter/farmer)

Most of the aged women who engage in traditional birth attendance practices and herbalists are held in high regard and esteem, as the people believe that their advice has kept the people from the evils of illnesses and death. One of the study participants, in her narrative, explained the reason the community has been standing behind the aged women and herbalists' practices.

> We have to turn to the practices of the elderly women, who are our mothers, and we have given birth over time, and to our fathers who turned herbalists and make use of roots and herbs, which we have in abundance here and are readily available to us without struggle. But the challenge is that only very few women can practice traditional birth attendance, and very few men have the gift of knowing which root or leaf can cure which disease. Therefore, we have to respect these few individuals and treat them with love because they have helped us, especially our children and women. (Pat, 40, farmer/trader)

Data gathered through discussions revealed that the farmers have turned to the hands of their aged mothers, who are forced into traditional birth-attendance practices by circumstances, and their fathers, who were also forced into herbalist practices due to the availability and accessibility of the roots and herbs within their settlement areas. The traditional birth attendants and herbalists were discovered to be working together with singleness of purpose, which is to save lives within the farm settlement area. Despite these community members taking to these alternative measures, most of the farmers still hold high hopes of health-care-intervention programmes for farmers in the farm settlement areas of AkwaIbom State.

DISCUSSION

The non-availability of maternal health-care services remains a serious challenge among the farmers in the Isohidim farm settlement area. This finding supports the position of Lassi, Salam, Das, and Bhutta (2014), who posit that poor maternal, newborn, and child health-care services have, over the decades, remained a visible health challenge among the low- and middle-income countries (LMICs), especially in sub-Saharan Africa. Interviews reveal the bitter experiences the farmers undergo due to the absence of maternal and reproductive health-care services. Study participants outlined their losses and the pain-bearing lifestyles of the women and children. In their lamentations, they narrated the loss of lives of women during labour and child mortality in the farm settlement areas, especially during child delivery, due to the absence of maternal health-care service providers and medical professionals or health workers in the Isohidim farm settlement community. This finding gives credence to the position of Izugbara, Wekesah, and Adedini (2016), who posit that, despite the global decline in maternal mortality since the 1990s, the maternal health experience continues to be risky for millions of Nigerian women, who have seen death and disability in many regions, states, communities in Nigeria. The finding also agrees with UNICEF (2009), that creating an enabling environment for safe motherhood and childbirth directly depends on the capacity to make available care and attention for pregnant women and their newborns in communities and families, the ability of skilled health workers, and the availability of adequate health-care facilities, equipment, and medicines and emergency care as when needed.

Information on the accessibility of maternal health-care services through interviews, discussions, and observations shows that most people in the Isohidim community do not have access to maternal and reproductive health care because of the absence of medical facilities in the farm settlement area under study. Only a few families who decided to access such care services were able to travel to other communities and neighbouring local government areas before they could get access to maternal health-care services. This situation has compounded the difficult experiences of the women and children living in the Isohidim community. These findings agree with the UNFPA (2013) report, that there are very few properly equipped health-care facilities in developing countries to take care of the maternal health care of women, and those that do exist are rarely capable of meeting the needs of the women and their babies. For some areas, like the farm settlement areas in AkwaIbom State, findings show there is a near-zero accessibility rate of maternal health care by farmers in the farm settlement areas.

On the utilization of alternative measures to maternal health-care services by farmers in the Isohidm farm settlement area, findings show that the farmers have, over the years, developed a dependency on the elderly women who have, over the years, gained experience in child delivery in the settlement areas, for maternal and reproductive care. Women of reproductive age have also gained a dependency on roots and herbs, and faith healing, for their health needs, due to the absence of medical health-care facilities to meet their maternal, reproductive, and other health needs. This dependency has generated bitter experiences for women and children, with a direct impact on families within the farm settlement areas. This finding agrees with Izugbara, Wekesah, and Adedini (2016), who further report that maternal health-care systems in Nigeria are in such a pathetic state that orthodox, faith-based, and traditional health providers, who are local injectionists, itinerant medicine hawkers, and patent medicine sellers have been gaining popularity. UNICEF (2009) also gives credence to the finding stating that many women in developing nations give birth at home without skilled or professional health-care workers present, yet their newborns are usually healthy and survive past their first few weeks of life, until their fifth birthdays, and despite the multitude of risks associated with pregnancy and childbirth, some of the mothers also survive although some lost their lives. The absence of maternal health-care services in the Isohidim farm settlement area has generated complicated and bitter experiences for the women of reproductive age and their children there.

CONCLUSION

Farm settlement areas are rural communities because they are always situated at the skirt of the urban centers. The people living in these farm settlement areas are referred to as the "poor class" because of their occupation and their socioeconomic status. Having realized their socioeconomic status, the farmers have decided to live within the context and capabilities of their social and economic definitions. The geo-location and socioeconomic status are responsible for the absence of maternal health-care services for the women of reproductive age who live there. In their quest for adaptation to their situation and to rescue their wives and children from a preventable death, the farmers have turned to the services of the aged women as traditional birth attendants (TBAs) and herbalists, who practice with root and herbs, and prayers for spiritual healings, which are easily available and accessible as alternatives to maternal and reproductive health-care services. The maternal health-care experiences of women of reproductive age in the Isohidim farm settlement area has become a fight against maternal and infant mortality. Based on the findings of the study, the researchers suggested the formulation of special health-care packages for farm settlement areas across the state, the provision of health-care centres in farm settlement areas by the local and state government, and government and non-governmental organizations undertaking health-care-intervention programmes for farmers in the farm settlements, especially for women and children, and finally, social amenities like good access roads and electricity being provided at the Isohidm and Akpansung communities in order to encourage people to bring health-care services to the areas.

REFERENCES

Fetterman, D. M. (2010). Ethnography: Step-by-Step. California: SAGE Publications, Inc., 42–50.

Izugbara, C.O., Wekesah, F. M., & Adedini, S. A. (2016). Maternal Health in Nigeria: A Situation Update. African Population and Health Research Center (APHRC), Nairobi, Kenya.

Lassi, Z. S., Salam, R. A., Das, J. A., & Bhutta, Z. A. (2014). Essential interventions for maternal, newborn and child health: background and methodology. *Reproductive Health Journal.* 11(Suppl 1):S1. http://www.reproductive-health-journal.com/content/11/S1/S1.

Okumagba, P. O. (2011). Choice of Health-Care Service Utilization by the Elderly in Delta State of Nigeria. *Journal of Sociology and Anthropology*, 2(2): 131–38.

Statista (2022). This Is How Africa Is Reducing Its Child Mortality Rate. Retrieved from https://www.weforum.org/agenda/2022/04/infant-mortality-africa-safer-future/ on 13 August 2022.

UNFPA (2013). Maternal Health Africa: Fact Sheet. https://www.unfpa.org/sites/default/files/resource-pdf/EN_Maternal%20Health%20in%20Africa_factsheet_web.pdf.

UNICEF (2009). Maternal and Newborn Health. https://www.unicef.org/media/84866/file/SOWC-2009.pdf.

WHO (2019). Maternal Mortality. https://www.who.int/news-room/fact-sheets/detail/maternal-mortality.

WHO (2022). Maternal Health. https://www.who.int/health-topics/maternal-health#tab=tab_1.

World Bank Group. (2016). Reproductive, Maternal, Newborn, and Child Health. https://openknowledge.worldbank.org/bitstream/handle/10986/23833/9781464803482.pdf.

Chapter 10

Socio-cultural Factors Affecting Menstrual Hygiene among Rural Women in the Anaang Communities of Akwa Ibom State, Nigeria

Nsidibe A. Usoro and Ursula V. Ette

INTRODUCTION

Despite the work done and the plethora of research conducted over the years of the past decades, in many African countries, reproductive health remains a key challenge (Frade, 2022). A systematic review of some literature that studied the link between water, sanitation hygiene, and maternal health in sub-Saharan Africa reported that water, sanitation, hygiene, and other extant socio-cultural factors were strongly associated with poorer maternal outcomes (Ononokpono, Baffour, Usoro, and Adeola, 2022). A study by Lahme et al. (2018) reported that the reproductive years of a woman are marked with many stages, and one of these is known as puberty. The onset of menstruation marks the stage of puberty, which continues throughout the reproductive years until the end, called menopause, which is the stage at which a woman is no longer menstruating.

Menstruation explains a physiological process through which a shedding of the uterine lining occurs each month in females of reproductive age (Derrick, Bryon, and Yafesi, 2017). Maintaining a good degree of hygiene during menstruation requires an adequate supply of and access to water.

It is commonplace that access to a safe and adequate water supply is key to maintaining good menstrual hygiene. Drinking water and using water for hygiene purposes are some of the high-priority needs of rural communities and households in Nigeria, since most of these poor communities are desirous of hygienic sources of water. Observations have shown that water management, provision, regulation, and distribution to end-users is, to a large extent, influenced by the behaviors and attitudes of people, which is strongly regulated by cultural practices, values, customs, and tradition in rural settings.

It is important to note that culture has an overbearing influence on humans in every society. Cultural practices are known to have the potential to regulate social activities and shape the interaction of people with their natural environment through rules and constraints. These informal constraints can often govern the success of formal constraints, which are established by scientific merit. Informal constraints are defined by day-to-day activities, while government and/or external agents introduce formal rules.

The challenge of accessibility to safe and hygienic menstrual-absorbent materials remains a significant setback, especially for girls from low socioeconomic backgrounds. A study by Boosey, Prestwich, and Deave (2014) reports that up to 87 percent of rural schoolgirls from western Uganda used old clothes or rags as menstrual absorbents, and yet these materials are infrequently changed, rarely washed with soap and clean water, and not properly dried prior to reuse. A similar study in rural western Kenya reveals that one in ten adolescents without access to sanitary pads also had no access to old cloths, mattress pieces, tissues, or other commonly cited menstrual-absorbent alternatives by girls in sub-Saharan Africa, owing to household impoverishment (Phillips-Howard, Otieno, Burmen, Otieno, Odongo, and Odour, 2015).

As a matter of fact, investigation has shown that most community infrastructure, for example in schools, lacks sufficient "girl-friendly" latrine facilities that maximize privacy, are clean and properly lit, are designed to accommodate girls with disabilities, and have flowing water and space for drying their menstrual-absorbent materials (Sommer, 2010). Available literature and studies have point to decaying or dearth of basic infrastructure to support WASH in most developing countries. In another study among Ethiopian schoolgirls, the authors reported that 85 percent of them did not change their menstrual soak-ups while at school, and 77 percent of the same categories of girls do not change their menstrual soak pads when at home (Derrick and Bryron, 2017). Over the last decades, many studies have been conducted on menstrual hygiene as a natural process, but most of these studies revolved around issues of poor management of menstruation by adolescent girls owing to their lack of skill and experience in handling menstruation, as well as any psychological demands that may arise during this delicate period. In many sub-Saharan Africa (SSA) rural communities, this normal process is considered taboo, and consequently, it is not discussed (Vaughehn, 2013).

The efficient management of menstruation by women in rural areas is hampered by a lack of knowledge and provision of other resources. Consequently, menstruation is often managed poorly and is often seen and described as an awkward, negative, and isolating experience by young girls of reproductive age.

Derick and Bryron (2017) identified poor access to dignified and functional water, sanitation, and hygiene (WASH) infrastructure in sub-Saharan Africa constitutes a major impediment for proper menstrual-hygiene management (MHM) within this region. There is no gain saying that improvement of MHM can contribute significantly towards the attainment of some of the sustainable development goals (SDG) mapped out in the United Nations Resolution: A/RES/70/1, including; (i) good health and well-being (SDG 3); (ii) inclusive and equitable quality education (SDG 4); (iii) gender equality and women's empowerment (SDG 5); (iv) clean water and sanitation (SDG 6); and (v) economic growth, productive employment and decent work for all (SDG 8). While there is obvious value for investing in MHM, few empirical studies on current knowledge, practices, and interventions for MHM among adolescent girls emanate from sub-Saharan Africa (Derick and Bryron, 2017).

THE CHALLENGES OF POOR MENSTRUAL HYGIENE

The poor and inefficient handling of sanitation and hygiene issues during menstruation militate against gender equity, and by extension, equitable quality education. To this end, some studies from sub-Saharan Africa estimate that between 50 and 70 percent of girls miss on average 1.6–2.1 days of school every month due to menstrual-related issues (Tegegne & Sisay, 2014; Boosey, Prestwich & Deave, 2014). Furthermore, many of those who manage to attend school during menstruation do so, but with low confidence and dignity, due to a disregard for their privacy, feelings of shame and embarrassment, in addition to the fear of being teased and bullied (Tegegne, Sisay, 2014). These authors further assert that these factors have been found to affect academic performance and to interfere with girls' participation in both school and extracurricular activities. The reality also is that most of the alternative absorbent materials used by girls in resource-poor households of rural communities are unsafe or used in unhygienic ways predisposes them to health risks that possibly underlie some common physiological complaints, such as vaginal pain, bruising, and reproductive-tract infections (Mason, Nyothach, Alexander, Odhiambo, Eleveld, and Vulule, 2013).

Other research, such as that conducted by Gultie, Hailu, and Workineh (2014), Gultie, Hailu, and Workineh (2015), and Mason, Nyothach, Alexander, Odhiambo, Eleveld, and Vulule (2013), argues that the failure to address menstrual-related needs is increasingly reported to result in prevalent risky sexual behavior. The occurrence of sex in exchange for money to buy sanitary pads and the dependency on boyfriends for sanitary pads is, for instance, reported in two studies among rural Kenyan adolescents.

INTERVENTIONS TO IMPROVE MENSTRUAL HYGIENE

Accessibility to physical infrastructure is the core of any intervention initiative, to lay the foundation stone upon which menstrual-hygiene management is built. These infrastructures are physical resources, such as WASH facilities and sanitary products, and the software components(education), that provide a knowledge-sharing platform that affects how women can leverage change and shape their behaviors to improve rhwie health outcomes (Montgomery, Ryus, Dolan, Dopson, and Scott, 2012; Sommer, 2016).

Sanitary products are either locally or commercially produced. Locally made products, like pads, are most preferable; this is in recognition of the fact that a number of cultural norms will not accept the insertion of a 'foreign object' into young girls (Derrick and Bryron, 2017). Besides being less affordable, commercial sanitary products have been reported to contribute to community waste (UNESCO, 2014). It should, however, be emphasized that despite creating new jobs in the community, the production of sanitary products may have a limited reach to consumers. According to Hennegan and Montgomery (2016), the provision of clean sanitary products has been hypothesized to reduce discomfort, as well as concerns regarding soiling outer garments during menstruation. The author went further to posit that improved management and comfort may also reduce the associated stigma and embarrassment that deters girls from attending school or work. There are already several local producers of sanitary products in African countries, such as AFRIpads (Uganda), Huru International (Kenya), and OneGirl (Sierra Leone), that focus on reusable, locally sourced, or low-cost sanitary products for girls and women in sub-Saharan Africa, or to teach them how to make their own reusable sanitary pads.

The utilization of such sustainable and inclusive innovations in health-care deliverables has the potential to boost economic activities and empowerment to some groups (i.e., adolescents and young women) and people from socio-economically disadvantaged backgrounds (Bitanihirwe, 2016).

Focusing on WASH facilities is another critical aspect of public health intervention. To achieve this end, it is important to develop a standard by which adolescents and young women are able to replace absorbents and wash their bodies in sex-segregated latrines in privacy, without attracting unwanted attention (UNESCO, 2014). Capacity building through an enlightenment campaign and education for girls and the wider community (i.e., boys and men) on menstruation is key to reducing the menace of discrimination and exclusion, because this initiative will surely create a supportive environment where women and girls can express their needs and emotions—particularly in contexts where there are significant taboos and restrictions, coupled with a lack of accurate information on sexual and reproductive health. Given the lack of awareness of menarche by many girls in sub-Saharan Africa, the stigma and taboos surrounding this topic has often prevented their access to accurate information to understand menstruation and its management (UNESCO, 2014).

Hennegan and Montgomery (2016) pointed out that better understanding and knowledge of MHM has been found to improve management practices, increase self-efficacy, and reduce anxiety and shame. It is recommended that puberty education begin in primary school so that girls understand what is happening to their bodies and know what to expect before menarche (UNESCO, 2014). This calls for a co-educational policy in which schools place emphasis on generating a curriculum that encourages respectful and understanding interpersonal relationships between boys and girls (Derrick and Bryron, 2017).

Menstrual periods call for deliberate actions and habits so as to appear neat and stay in a clean environment. Many precautionary or intervention activities should be carried out to improve the sanitary conditions of a woman during her menstrual period; this is called menstrual hygiene.

Menstrual hygiene in women requires using clean menstrual materials to absorb or collect menstrual blood, which can be changed in privacy as often as necessary for the duration of a menstrual period, as well as using soap and water for washing the body as required and having access to safe and convenient facilities to dispose of used menstrual materials.

Menstrual hygiene practice is as old as humans have been in existence (Derrick et.al., 2017), and it requires a deliberate effort to maintain a high level of cleanliness and other healthy habits by women during their menstrual period. Women everywhere hope to appear neat and decent throughout their periods and prevent infectious diseases spread especially through uncleanliness during the period.

Menstrual periods must be handled with care, and the best available hygiene practices to avoid or reduce vulnerability to infections during the period should be used, as doing otherwise could lead to serious health issues, such as infertility and other damaging maternal health conditions.

Global Health Promotion (2019) has stated that maximizing menstrual-hygiene interventions calls for deliberate actions to identify hygiene needs; the integration of both knowledge and skill training gained through education on menstrual hygiene management (MHM); in addition to the improvement of access to girl-friendly water, sanitation, and hygiene facilities, as well as access to low-cost hygienic sanitary products. To facilitate the identification and implementation of feasible and cultural relevant programs, we recommend the utilization of public-health-intervention research. This provision serves as a major inspiration for the coinage of the theme for 2016's World Population Day, which was 'investing in teenage girls.'

The foregoing suggests that findings from multiple studies illustrate that many negative feelings related to MHM are tied to the notion of menstruation being associated with sexual impurity (Vaughn, 2013). In Nigeria, particularly in the rural villages, this notion is the cause of a culture of silence and shame surrounding issues associated with sexuality and menstruation (Onyegegbu, 2011). In Kenya, girls express concern about being stigmatized by fellow students due to the cultural belief that menarche signals the advent of a girl's sexual status (McMahon, Winch, Caruso, Obure, Ogutu, and Ochari, 2011). In Tanzania, many girls do not disclose to anyone when they initiate menarche, because it is believed to be associated with improper sexual behavior; they fear they will be accused of premarital sexual activity. Consequently, over half of the rural respondents from the Tanzanian study claim to have disclosed their "secret" for the first time to the researchers (Sommer, 2011).

Schoolgirls report that their challenges during menstruation related to hygiene, leakages, and insufficient privacy are often the cause of embarrassment and stigma. Some teachers suppose that girls who accidentally stain their uniforms during menstruation are "misbehaving." This supposition demonstrates the offense of the social taboo (Crichton, Okal, Kabiru, and Zulu, 2012). Girls communicate feeling anxious constantly during their menses, owing to fear of leakage and body odor due to infrequent changing of their menstrual hygiene products. Girls report being bullied if their peers at schools discover they are menstruating. Sometimes boys suspect that a girl is menstruating when she wears a sweater around her waist or if it smells like she "killed a chicken" (Matovu, 2011).

Male perceptions of menstruation are often driven by stereotypical notions and lack of knowledge about menstruation. Ignorance about menstruation only increases the negative expressions and teasing, particularly from boys to girls. Girls express that the fear of ridicule decreases their confidence levels at school (Matovu, 2011).

The lack of knowledge and education about menstruation feeds into many traditional beliefs and cultural practices that exacerbate the negative feelings many schoolgirls experience, since these beliefs and practices often lead girls to feel isolated and stigmatized, as well as discourage girls from participating in school and other social events while menstruating (Vaughn, 2013).

Women in rural communities suffer more from restrictions, marginalization, and isolation because of strict adherence to the social and cultural norms and values handed over to them by their ancestors in the aspects of respect to elders and husbands. Some of these have become repulsive, outdated, and awkward, without any sane logic in modern times. This study is a qualitative exploration of some cultural factors underlying the knowledge of menstrual hygiene management among rural Anaang women, with the specific objectives of identifying the local absorbent materials used by rural women in the area and their effect on MHM.

Many researchers in this area of study were not too eager to explore the interference of socio-cultural factors on menstrual-hygiene management in developing societies. Recognizing this gap in research, this study, through rapid key informant investigation and community conversations with women of reproductive age, aims to inform the understanding of some entangling web of socio-cultural factors militating against effective menstrual-hygiene management.

MATERIAL AND METHODS

A multi-sited qualitative exploration of competing narratives were conducted in three Anaang-speaking communities (Ika,Ikot, Obio Akpa, and Ebebit Afaha Obong). Anaang people are found in Akwa Ibom State, south of Nigeria. They are the second-largest ethnic group of the state, occupying its northern part. They are bounded in the north by Isogbo Igbo (Abia State), in the west by the *Ngwas* and *Ndoki* (Abia State), and in the southeast and northeast by the *Ibibios.* Anaang is a patrilineal society. The people speak *Anaang* as a language and have great respect for the elders as required by their culture and tradition (Usoro and Ekong, 2016). The people traditionally worship *Akwa Awashi Ibom* (the Almighty God). Their natural resources include palm fruits; they are large producers of palm oil. Their occupation is mainly farming and petty trading.

Information used in this study was collected through rapid key informant interviews (RKII) and community conversation sessions (CCS). One hundred and fifty (150) women were conveniently recruited from three Anaang communities (Ika,Ikot, Obio Akpa, and Ebebit Afaha Obong) in Nigeria were interviewed in early 2021.These locations were chosen for the interview due to their rural settings. Purposive sampling was used to ensure that only women of reproductive age were recruited to participate in the in-depth interview exercise.

All women enlisted for the study were willing to participate, and written consent was obtained from each participant; those who could not fill out the consent form were assisted by field assistants. The inclusion criteria were women aged between the ages of fourteen and forty-nine years who have seen menses. Light refreshments and honorariums were given to participants as a way of appreciating them for their time.

RESULTS

Responses to qualitative interviews and community conversation sessions were recorded from the study locations and thematically presented in perspectives. A few of the participants were professionals, such as teachers and health workers, while the majority were peasant farmers, petty traders, and housewives. Excerpts presented here are raw narratives from participants during RKII and CCS.

Socio-Demographic Information

The mean age of participants during community conversation was forty-six years. All discussants were women of reproductive age who have ever experienced menarche. RKII respondents had a mean age of forty-two years. Out of the 180 respondents, 150 respondents were females, while the remaining thirty were males. Available statistics revealed that fifty discussants participated in CCS, and they were all women randomly drawn from all walks of life in the study communities. Twenty (20) out the fifty discussants were educated beyond the primary-school level. Also, fifty out of the 130 respondents interviewed attended school beyond the primary/standard-six level.

Knowledge of Menstrual Hygiene Management

All participants knew of menstruation, locally known as *Itie isong* (sitting on the bare floor or ground), *Nkut Enang* (seeing the cow), *or Mbiomo* idem (body burden), and they claimed to have experienced menarche. The study participants noted that their information/knowledge of managing menstrual hygiene was handed down to them by mothers and elders in the communities. They noted generally that the menstrual period requires deliberate attention to ensure personal hygiene and sanitation of the environment. They identified water as a very essential need in an effective menstrual-hygiene-management system. Local reusable materials, such as pieces of cloth, towels and wrappers, banana fibers, soft leaves, and cotton wool, were used for managing hygiene. Modern absorbent materials, such as sanitary pads, tampons, toilet tissue, and a menstrual cup, were used by those who could afford them. A majority of discussants and interview respondents pointed out:

Information about proper menstrual-hygiene management was not available in those days. We were basically told and shown how to apply the local reusable materials, like torn wrappers, pieces of cloth, and towels to absorb the blood by our mothers and elderly women close to us. These were disposed of at the nearby surroundings. No special consideration was given to women under menses where there is an acute shortage of water in the community.

My mother was the first person who used to tell me about menstruation. When I finally experienced it, she followed me to the bathroom and showed me how to clean myself properly, and how to fold and insert the piece of cloth to absorb the blood.

As young girls, we used to share information given to us by our parents among us. But this discussion were always in low tones and when the boys were not around. I was always shy, timid, and ashamed of myself during my period.

My mother told me to always wash the cloth properly and keep it inside a special cellophane bag for reuse. We were also advised to keep a safe distance from public gatherings to prevent people from perceiving the faint odor of the blood flow. I normally used sanitary pads and sometimes toilet tissue to collect the flows.

When I am menstruating, I make sure there is enough water to have regular baths and wash my undies and other reusable absorbent materials. A hot bath was recommended by my mother during this period, and I strictly adhered to this.

I normally used sanitary pads to absorb the blood during my menses. But there was a time when I tried out a menstrual cup. (Probing further . . .) A menstrual cup is used to collect menstruation; it is a small elastic cup inserted inside the vagina to collect the blood. It is designed with a little ropelike tip to pull it out after some hours of use. I was introduced to it in Lagos when I visited my aunt.

Socio-Cultural Factors Influencing Menstrual Hygiene in the Rural Anaang Community

Participants in interviews reported marginalization, poor socioeconomic status, ignorance, influence of the elderly, environmental factors, cultural beliefs and values, misconceptions and myths, and socio-cultural factors that influenced their menstrual-hygiene management in the study area.

Issues of Marginalization

Anaang is a patrilineal society, and social interactions and the value system accord men the right to dominate and feel superior over women. The participants reported that gender-specific issues affecting only the women attract little or no attention. Access and availability of water for household use poses serious challenges, especially where women depend on men for water, because cultural belief forbids women who experience menstruation to enter and fetch water in the village streams. There are also reports of cases where customs and traditions regard women experiencing menstruation as unclean, and therefore, unfit to cook or sleep with their husbands; they were also excluded from partaking in many other cultural rites. This turn of events highlights issues of gender equity and marginalization of women. Even the local terminologies used in describing menstruation in the Anaang lexicon—*itie isong*—literally means "sitting on the floor or ground"; *Mbiomo Idem* ("body burden"), and *Nkut Enang* ("seeing the beast of burden"). These serve to dwindle the social status of women during menstruation. So many women interviewed reported many cases of marginalization due to the sense of shame, segregation, and inferiority imposed on them by the patrilineal nature of the society (RKII& CCS):

> Because of my menses, I am forbidden from going to fetch water from our village stream; it is my husband and children that do this, and the water is not always enough for domestic and my personal use during sanitation. I feel deprived because it is my husband alone who determined the amount of water available in the house and therefore the quantity I can use.
>
> We always have this horrible sense of inferiority when we are restricted or excluded from living our normal lives, simply because of having monthly flows. It makes us feel abnormal or that maybe something is wrong with us, whereas we are as normal as every other person in this community.
>
> As women, we are expected to discharge our cultural motherly responsibilities, such as cooking, caring, and other domestic chores, without discrimination. But immediately when menstruation sets in, we were isolated and regarded as socially unclean to interact and do certain things in this community.
>
> My husband does accept food from me. . . . We hug and play with each other, but he declines actual lovemaking even when I need it, claiming that it is a taboo to have sex with a woman experiencing menstruation.

> I continue to live my normal life. . . . I cook for my husband when I am menstruating. We have managed to live above some cultural values that do not appeal to modern-day reality.

> In the olden days, there were so many restrictions against the women in this community, and having sex with a woman experiencing menstruation was a taboo. But now, with the advent of Christianity, people are beginning to see things differently. To me it is superstitious to believe that somebody is impure because she is menstruating.

Factors Related to Socioeconomic Status

Some women reported they do not have enough money to care for themselves and provide food for their families; hence, they have an inability to buy sanitary napkins or pads or towels during menstruation. This has made them resort to using old torn wrappers/cloths, which are washed, dried, and kept for reuse the next month. Participants narrated (RKII&CCS):

> We do not have money for sanitary pads, so my husband advised me to use my torn wrappers during menses. I wash the cloth and preserve it for reuse in the future. We are poor here, and the little income is not even enough to feed our children and care for other important needs. The majority of us are housewives with a meager income from menial jobs, the willingness to use sanitary pads may be there, but the money is not available.

> The village stream and ponds had dried up. The only source of water was a private borehole, which you have to pay for. I had to manage the little water we could afford to clean myself and for domestic use.

> Whenever I cannot afford the cost of sanitary pads, I use my torn wrappers to collect the flow, which I wash, dry, and reuse in the future until the piece of cloth is completely worn out. Women in this community used banana fibers and soft leaves to collect the blood in those days.

Poor Knowledge of Modern Menstrual Hygiene

Most of the rural women of these communities do not know the implications of using unhygienic materials, as their main concern is what can absorb the blood without other people knowing that she is experiencing menstruation. The study participants reported:

> My late mother taught me how to manage menstruation using local materials, such as rags or torn wrappers to collect the bleeding. We were also advised to

eat plenty of pepper to quicken the process. In those days, there were no pads or other modern technologies developed to manage menstrual periods.

Although there was advice on personal hygiene during menstruation, the extent of our hygiene was dependent on the availability of water. I was not aware of the importance of water, sanitation, and hygiene (WASH), and the fact that poor menstrual-hygiene management could lead to serious health issues was not emphasized.

Influence of the Elderly

The women acknowledged that *menses* is defined within the lexicon of taboo language that young people are not allowed to mention in public. Therefore, the younger women rely on the elderly for interpretation, advice, and intervention during times of menstruation. According to the participants (RKII&CCS):

> Hmm . . . my son, in those days nobody mentioned menses in the public, as it connotes embarrassment and shame. Young people talked about it with hushed voices; therefore, all issues associated with it were directed to the elderly women for guidance and advice.

> Menstruation management, and other challenges associated with it, are not just private issues, but are treated as sacred discussions where only the elderly people have the exclusive right to inform the community. Therefore, the manner and how to manage menstruation hygiene were determined by the elderly women.

> In the olden days, even in present times, many young girls who experienced menstruation for the first time felt more comfortable to confide in their mothers or any other available elderly person for advice on how to manage the condition.

Environmental Factors

The communities' lack of a good water supply or a natural source of water that is clean makes it difficult for the people to have access to water where and when it is necessary. Also, the people use pit toilets—some with or without a covering—as well as makeshift bathrooms, which provide less privacy, hence their inability to properly attend to their personal hygiene. According to the participants (CCS):

> We do not have adequate source of water supply in this community. The only stream we have is far away at the outskirts of the community, and it is mixed with a clay substance that makes it not good for drinking and hygiene purposes.

> As you can observe, we have predominantly pit toilets in this community. That's our makeshift bathroom over there. They are shared . . . only a few people can afford self-contained apartments.

> The facility for hygiene is not adequate. Apart from not looking good, sometimes, especially in the morning when you are inside the bathroom, you find out that so many other people are also waiting. So you just rush out to avoid conflict with people.

Cultural Beliefs and Values

The women are culturally expected to be submissive and obedient to all laws of the land. They are not to enter the stream during their menses so that the source of water will not be polluted, as they are culturally seen as being unclean. A participant said (RKII):

> Yes, here is the general belief that menstruating women carry an antidote, and as such are prevented from attending certain traditional functions, as well as passing through some places such as the Shrine Village Square (Afe or Anwa Isong) so that the powers there will not be neutralized.

> Menstruation was often considered a taboo subject; menstruation is seldom openly discussed in this community. People who dared to discuss it openly were condemned as being irresponsible and deviants in the society.

> Young people who discussed issues relating to menstruation were seen as lacking in proper upbringing and were seriously reprimanded and sometimes beaten to serve as a deterrent to others.

Misconceptions and Myths

It was believed that menstruation is a secret thing among women and that no one should ever know when a woman is menstruating. Also, the use of pads/sanitary towels was not advised, as it is believed that people can carry them and use them for diabolical things that can render them infertile. Some participants narrated (CCS):

> It is not advisable to disclose your menstruation status to people who are not close or trustworthy. There was this fear that evil people could manipulate the condition to cause infertility issues to the woman in the future, by having access to any item she used in managing her hygiene during the period.

> We were told not to display or dry the wrappers or other items we used to pack ourselves outside to avoid being contaminated by the evil spirits. Also, the use of modern sanitary pads was regarded with suspicion; no one was encouraged to insert any foreign materials into her private parts . . . in those days.
>
> It was believed that women who had their menses were possessed by certain spirits that could neutralize protective charms and amulets and destroy their efficacy. It was also believed that people who had sex with women who were experiencing menstruation would contract an infection and eventually die.

Effects of Poor Menstrual Hygiene

Observations and available facts revealed that a poor perception of menstruation provided the seedbed for mishandling menstrual-hygiene processes in the study area. Since the menstrual period is one of the major issues of stigmatization, young girls view menarche as the onset of a monthly period of shame, isolation, and restricted freedoms. Women were not free to discuss menses-related issues publicly. Women were oriented to bear this condition in silence as the price to be paid for womanhood. This culture of silence made some women conceal menstruation-related health issues that needed urgent medical attention. Consequently, there were incidents of serious health complications, such as tubal blockage, infections of hepatitis B, vulva scabies, and other, fatal cases. The study participants reported (RKII&CCS):

> We had cases where some women complained of irregular or scanty blood flows, and some even complained of complete stoppage. These challenges and many others could be connected to poor management of one's menstruation period.
>
> We lost a certain woman in this community last week who became seriously sick; after all efforts to cure her with local herbs failed, she was taken to the hospital, where the doctor said she was suffering from infections because the monthly flow of her menses had been blocked. Many other women have gone the same way. Some were diagnosed with hepatitis B and vulva scabies.
>
> Neglecting to wash hands after changing menstrual products due to a lack of water can spread infections such as hepatitis B and thrush. The use of unhygienic/infected materials can also result in vulvar scabies.
>
> I do not quickly discuss health issues relating to my menses with people, especially those of the opposite sex, because of shame. Even when I go to the clinic, I find it difficult to open up to a male physician. It is not my fault—that is how I was brought up.

DISCUSSION

Evidence from the study points to the fact that rural women only prepared the minds of their daughters about menarche, but they failed to impart proper knowledge of menstrual-hygiene management. Arguably, the majority of mothers lack correct information to pass on to their daughters in this regard. Studies suggest that women in rural communities communicate with their girls about the onset of menstruation by preparing a special food for her and the rest of the house, then passing on warnings about staying away from boys and about pregnancy risks (Onyegegbu, 2011). Often these messages are delivered in harsh tones, and sometimes false information is passed along. Other families secretly rejoice when a daughter matures to womanhood. When probed further about discussing menstruation with their daughters, the women convey they often impart traditional practices and knowledge they learned from their own mothers. Some mothers believe it is important to talk to their daughters about menstruation, and they would like to be able to share biological information about menstruation (Onyegegbu, 2011).

Discussions and interviews of participants revealed that women were isolated and restricted from doing certain things or going to certain places during their menses. In some horrible cases, they are not allowed even to access the village stream or to cook for their husbands. A situation where only the male will fetch water for the house gave the men more power or rights over the water than the women. This can result in conflict, a seedbed for domestic violence in which the women are the most vulnerable. The various local terms used in describing menstruation, such as *itie isong* (literally meaning "sitting on the floor or bare ground"); *Mbiomo Idem* ("body burden"); and *Nkut Enang* ("seeing the beast of burden"), are suggestive of the debased status of women in the study area. This turn of events has exacerbated gender inequality in the study setting.

As at the twenty-first century, millions of women and girls around the world are being stigmatized, excluded and discriminated against, and isolated, and they are viewed as something dirty or filthy and unhealthy, thereby requiring restrictions from certain activities due to menstruation—which is simply a natural bodily function (Ekane, Nykvist, Kjellén, Noel, and Weitz , 2014).

Derrick et al. (2017) submits that improvement of MHM contributed immensely towards the achievement of a number of sustainable development goals (SDG) contained in the United Nations Resolution: A/RES/70/1, including (i) good health and well-being (SDG 3); (ii) inclusive and equitable quality education (SDG 4); (iii) gender equality and women's empowerment (SDG 5); (iv) clean water and sanitation (SDG 6); and (v) economic growth, productive employment, and decent work for all (SDG 8). Although the value for investing in menstrual-hygiene management is obvious, there exist few empirical studies on current knowledge, practices, and interventions for MHM among adolescent girls that emanate from sub-Saharan Africa.

Menstrual hygiene is one of the critical health issues affected by some socio-cultural factors in many developing countries of the world, and the consequences of poor menstrual practice everywhere in the world have the potential to aggravate the myriads of maternal health issues among women in such societies.

Poverty, ignorance, undue paternal influence, cultural beliefs, misconceptions/myths, and environmental factors were identified by study participants as key variables influencing menstrual-hygiene management. Menstruation is still considered a taboo that cuts across various cultures, and both old and young women of some communities feel that menstruation is a curse or a burden (Ekane et al., 2014). Global Health Promotion (2019) stipulates that maximizing menstrual-hygiene interventions calls for deliberate actions to identify hygiene needs; integration of both knowledge and skill/training gained through education on menstrual hygiene management (MHM)' in addition to improvement of access to girl-friendly water, sanitation, and hygiene facilities, as well as access to low-cost hygienic sanitary products.

Across the globe, sub-Saharan Africa (SSA) has been observed to be home to one of the world's fastest-growing teenage-girl populations (Population Reference Bureau. 2013), a majority of whom will or already have had the onset of menstruation (menarche). Despite the fact that menstruation is a natural human-developmental process, government sectors, such as health and education departments in developing countries, are not eager or keen at prioritizing issues related to it (UNESCO, 2014). For young girls of reproductive age, the menstrual period may come with various challenges, owing to poor management of menstrual hygiene, the lack of disposable income to access menstrual-absorbent materials, and the psychological demands they experience during this delicate period of change (UNESCO, 2014). Moreover, poor access to dignified and functional water, sanitation, and hygiene (WASH) infrastructure in developing countries around African continents (Ekane, Nykvist, Kjellén, Noel, and Weitz, 2014) remains a major setback for the effective management of menstrual hygiene by adolescent girls within this region.

CONCLUSION

Menstrual-hygiene management is a critical human-rights issue that impacts social and economic rights, including health, water, sanitation, education, and work. Extant literature reviewed in this study points at myriads of topical issues posed by the problem to governments, donor agencies, and public health bodies. This study represents one of the high-quality studies that focuses on providing a qualitative exploration of competing narratives regarding MHM in the study area.

This study made a strong case for capacity building through an enlightenment campaign and education for girls and other critical stakeholders in the wider community (such as boys and men) on menstruation, as key to reducing the menace of discrimination and exclusion. It is the position of this study that this kind of initiative is needed to galvanize a supportive environment where women and girls can express their needs and emotions without undue influence by cultural practices and belief systems, such as taboos, customs, values, and its attendant restrictions. Accurate information on sexual and reproductive health is also a very critical consideration.

Socioeconomic factors, such as poor socioeconomic status, ignorance, the influence of the elderly, cultural beliefs and values, misconceptions, and myths, generate reasonable impacts towards the current MHM-related barriers facing women of reproductive age in the study area, changes are required in terms of women's education regarding their reproductive health, the environmental impact through the appropriate disposal of menstrual waste, and the production, marketing, and accessibility of low-cost sanitary products. Together, these initiatives will help demystify taboos around menstruation and empower girls and women.

Cultural responses to issues associated with menstrual hygiene are unique, based on educational levels, income levels, and exposure to modern hygiene facilities or technologies. In this case, no uniform intervention may successfully address the poor management of menstrual hygiene among the study population. Therefore, this study lends its voice to the call for broad-based programmatic public health intervention policies with key emphases on an increasing-awareness campaign on proper menstrual hygiene practices; the provision of social amenities such as good water supplies and toiletries; in addition to creating and maintaining a good cultural environment to manage menstruation conditions with a high degree of hygiene and human dignity. Above all, an education policy that incorporates MHM in school curriculum will help to dismiss misconceptions and superstitions, build the capacity for and boost the confidence of young girls approaching menarche to confront the process with adequate hygiene-management skills. These suggestions will be of key significance in addressing the substantial issues of concern raised in this area of study.

REFERENCES

Bitanihirwe, B.K. (2016). Scaling-up innovation as a means of tackling health inequalities. *Ann Ist Super Sanita,* 52: 143–45.

Boosey, R., Prestwich, G., and Deave, T. (2014). Menstrual hygiene management amongst schoolgirls in the Rukungiri district of Uganda and the impact on their education: a cross-sectional study. *Pan Afr Med J.,* 19: 253.

Derrick, S., and Bryron, K. (2017). Menstrual Hygiene Management among Adolescent Girls in Sub-Saharan Africa. *Global Health Promotion,*1757–9759, vol. 26(1): 105–08;694597.

Ekane, N., Nykvist, B., Kjellén, M., Noel, S., Weitz, N. (2014). Multi-level sanitation governance: understanding and overcoming challenges in the sanitation sector in sub-Saharan Africa. *Waterlines,* 33:242–56.

Frade, S. (2022). *From post-colonialism to Cairo to now: The (u)changing ideas of reproductive health and family planning in Africa.* In Odimegwu &Adewoyin (eds). *The Routledge Handbook of African Demography.* London and New York: Taylor and Francis Group.

Gultie, T., Hailu, D., Workineh, Y. (2014). Age of menarche and knowledge about menstrual hygiene management among adolescent schoolgirls in Amhara province, Ethiopia: implication to health care workers & schoolteachers. *PLoS One,* 9: e108644.

Hawe, P., Potvin, L. (2009). What is population health intervention research? *Journal of Public Health,* 2 100: 8–14.

Hennegan, J., Montgomery, P. (2016). Do menstrual hygiene management interventions improve education and psychosocial outcomes for women and girls in low- and middle-income countries? a systematic review. *PLoS One*, 11: e0146985. *J R Soc Health,* 1986; 106: 219–21.

Lahme, A.M., Stern, R., Cooper, D. (2016). Factors impacting on menstrual hygiene and their implications for health promotion. *Glob Health Promot.* DOI: 10.1177/1757975916648301.

Lawan, U.M., Yusuf, N.W., Musa, A.B. (2010). Menstruation and menstrual hygiene amongst adolescent schoolgirls in Kano, Northwestern Nigeria. *African Journal of Reproductive Health,* 14: 201–07.

Mason, L., Nyothach, E., Alexander, K., Odhiambo, F.O., Eleveld, A., and Vulule, J. (2013). 'We keep it secret so no one should know'—a qualitative study to explore young schoolgirls attitudes and experiences with menstruation in rural western Kenya. *PLoS One,* 8: e79132.

Matovu, N.F. (2011). *Pubescent girls' menstrual experiences and implications for their schooling: a Ugandan case study* [master's thesis]. International Institute of Graduate Studies. http://oaithesis.eur.nl.libproxy.lib.unc.edu/ir/repub/asset/10851 /Nalubega_Fatuma_Matovu_Final_RP_submission.docx (accessed January 20, 2013).

McMahon, S., Winch, P., Caruso, B., Obure, A., Ogutu, E., Ochari, I. (2011). "The girl with her period is the one to hang her head": Reflections on menstrual management among schoolgirls in rural Kenya. *BMC Int Health Hum Rights*, 11(1): 7. http:

//www.doaj.org.libproxy.lib.unc.edu/doaj?func=abstract&id=796874 (accessed February 4, 2013).

Montgomery, P., Ryus, C.R., Dolan, C.S, Dopson, S., Scott, L.M. (2012). Sanitary pad interventions for girls' education in Ghana: a pilot study. *PLoS One*, 7: e48274.

Ononokpono, D.N., Baffour, B., Usoro, N., and Adebola, O. (2022). *Maternal mortality in sub-Saharan Africa: Systematic review of measurement, levels and determinants*. In Odimegwu & Adewoyin (eds).*The Routledge Handbook of African Demography.* London and New York: Taylor and Francis Group.

Onyegegbu, N. (2011). Menstruation and menstrual hygiene among women and young females in rural eastern Nigeria. *Journal of the Science Teachers Association of Nigeria.* http://stanonline.org/journal/pdf/JSTAN-Nkadi%202011.pdf (accessed February 4, 2013).

Osujih, M. (1986). Menstruation problems in Nigerian students and sex education. *J R.Soc Health,* 106: 219–21.

Phillips-Howard, P.A., Otieno, G., Burmen, B., Otieno, F., Odongo, F., and Odour, C. (2015). Menstrual needs and associations with sexual and reproductive risks in rural Kenyan females: a cross-sectional behavioral survey linked with HIV prevalence. *Journal of Women Health*, 24: 801–11.

Population Reference Bureau. (2013). *World Population Data Sheet.* Washington, DC: Population Reference Bureau, 2013.

Sahin, M., Joshi, D., Buit, G., and González-Botero, D. (2015). Menstrual hygiene management: education and empowerment for girls? *Waterlines,* 34: 51–67.

Skumani. (2017). "Social, Cultural and religious practices during menstruation." *Jharkhad Journal of Development and Management Studies* XISS, Ranchi, Vol. 15 (2017).

Sommer, M., Caruso, B.A., Sahin, M., Calderon, T., Cavill, S., and Mahon, T. (2016). A time for global action: addressing girls' menstrual hygiene management needs in schools. *PLoS Med.,* 13: e1001962.

Sommer, M. (2010). Putting menstrual hygiene management on to the school water and sanitation agenda. *Waterlines,* 29: 268–78.

Sommer, M. (2011). An early window of opportunity for promoting girls' health: policy implications of the girl's puberty book project in Tanzania. *Int Electron J Health Educ*., 14: 77–92. http://growandknow.org/11_M-Sommer.pdf (accessed 20 January 2013).

Tegegne, T.K., Sisay, M.M. (2014). Menstrual hygiene management and school absenteeism among female adolescent students in Northeast Ethiopia. *BMC Public Health,* 14: 1118.

UNESCO. (2014). *Good policy and practice in health education.* Booklet 9. Puberty Education & Menstrual Hygiene Management. Paris, France: UNESCO; 2014.

Upashe, S.P., Tekelab, T., Mekonnen, J. (2015). Assessment of knowledge and practice of menstrual hygiene among high school girls in Western Ethiopia. *BMC Women's Health,* 15: 84.

Usoro, N.A., and Ekong, I.C. (2016). The place of cultural realities and symbolic forms among Anaang people of Akwa Ibom State, Nigeria. *South-South Journal of Culture and Development*, 18(1): 122–40.

Vaughan, J.G. (2013). *A review of menstrual hygiene management among schoolgirls in Sub-Saharan Africa.* A paper presented to the faculty of the University of North Carolina at Chapel Hill.

Chapter 11

Socio-Economic and Health Assessment of Internally Displaced Persons in North East Nigeria

Mohammed Saeed Suleiman

INTRODUCTION

Nigeria as a country is faced with the challenges of internally displaced persons (IDPs) that continues to generate global concern owing to its negative implications on the socioeconomic and health structure of the society. Globally, it is observed that the regulation on human rights speculates the rights of all and sundry to gain from acceptable housing, social security, and a good standard of living as noted by the United Nations [UN] (2018), that the right to ample housing provision includes protection against forced evictions, arbitrary demolition or pulling down of one's home, confidentiality, and family, to select one's residence or determine where to live, and freedom of movement. It is observed that in spite of the different international and national human rights law that seeks to guarantee a healthy and unprejudiced environment, and pleasant atmosphere for mankind, the major force behind human displacement has been ascribed to large-scale natural disasters and armed human conflicts, which for the developing nations are worse, affected by unplanned human displacement as noted by Umar, Suleiman, and Magaji (2018) that Nigeria as a state recently remains besieged in internal insurgencies ranging from different types of the uprising and resulting in the flow of thousands of IDPs from one area to another and by implication living as marginal communities in sub-Saharan Africa.

The preceding studies have shown that in sub-Saharan Africa, several preventable challenges and insurgencies are frequently linked to human direct or indirect dealings that frighten human habitation and by implication lead to the increasing number of IDPs globally. ss observed by Kevin (2018), Africa as a continent is horrible concerning the IDPs, and the region keeps on to witness the rising figure of IDPs, notwithstanding the efforts to have this occurrence mitigated. The United Nations Refugee Agency [UNHCR] (2017) posits that the predominance of forced IDPs was about 68.5 million individuals globally, owing to different factors such as insurgencies, economic hardship, and natural disasters, among others. With the emergence of the Boko Haram insurgency (BHI), Nigeria has the highest number of IDPs, as observed by the Norwegian Refugee Council (NRC)(2017). The BHI incident has forced many people to flee their homes, and consequently Nigeria has become a nation with the maximum figure of IDPs in sub-Saharan Africa. Similarly, in Nigeria, women and children form the highest number of IDPs, as noted by the Displacement Tracking Matrix (DTM)(2017). Women and children account for 79 percent of the IDP population, and children less than five years old account for 28 percent of the population. Similarly, this study observed that displaced women and girls have been the worse hit concerning having accessibility to fundamental rights and health services, as well as gender-based violence in camps repeatedly weakening long-lasting solutions. Thus, the surfacing of insurgencies has occurred, especially Boko Haram; this has become a recurrent issue accompanied by socioeconomic and health burdens and implications. The IDPs are considered marginal communities in sub-Saharan Africa.

In the context of literature and marginality, Bhagwan (2013) expressed that internal displacement interrupts the socioeconomic activities and structures of the areas left behind and the people flee to these IDPs. Similarly, IDPs are mostly large in number and susceptible in nature to compete with the host communities in the utilization of the available limited resources. By implication, this can lead to poor living conditions or conflict because the available scarce resources can hardly cater to the needs of all the people. As advanced by Asphlet (2013), internal displacement happens on a substantial scale and by implication; the migration of IDPs into an area can dislocate the complete region, particularly when the particular region is not prepared or has fewer resources to cater to the influx of the IDPs. To this end, IDPs face psychological trauma, which makes them vulnerable to human rights abuses, poor living conditions, and poor health care, among others. Thus, this study sees IDPs as marginal communities in sub-Saharan Africa. Similarly, IDPs are faced with the challenges of poor accessibility to food, nutrition, health care, shelter, water, sanitation, and education, among others, as pointed out by the United Nations Office for the Coordination of Humanitarian Affairs (UNOCHA)

(2018). IDPs in northeast Nigeria are in serious need of life-saving support such as food and nutrition, health care, shelter, non-food items, potable water, and improved sanitation and hygiene conditions. This study observed that IDPs are living as marginal communities in sub-Saharan Africa.

Thus, the objective of this study is to investigate and bring to the forefront the socioeconomic and health assessments of IDPs in northeast Nigeria. The chapter also attempts to contribute to the academic literature despite the amount of research that has been conducted in this area. In addition, a review of literature posits that the challenges of IDPs have continued to generate global concern because of their negative implications on the socioeconomic and health structures of the society, with severe deprivation, hardship, and discrimination, among others. It is against this background that this chapter raised the question that despite all the efforts put in place by the government and humanitarian organizations to address the challenges of IDPs, the socio-economic and health conditions of IDPs in the northeast are still unbearable and they provoke the deteriorating living conditions of the IDPs, who are living as marginal communities in sub-Saharan Africa.

This study adopts two theories: the forced migration theory and the social inclusion theory. However, this is not to undermine other theoretical constructs that have been used to explain the phenomenon under review. The trends of IDPs are alarming, as a result of forced displacement arising from natural and environmental disasters, as well as violence and armed conflict as it applies to the IDPs in northeast, Nigeria. It is pertinent to mention that forced migration entails the involuntary movement of people from their places of accustomed residence due to happenings threatening the safety of their lives (Benz and Hasenclever, 2009). Thus, forced migration theory vividly elucidates the increase of involuntary movement of people with the harsh conditions IDPs strive for a living as related to the plights of IDPs in the northeast. IDPs can be described as individuals who have been forcefully ejected from their places of dwelling and with the fear that the government failed to curb the menaces of the rebellious activities of severe deprivation, hardship, psychological trauma, and discrimination, among others. These have continued to affect the lives and property of the IDPs, as advanced by Castles (2009) such that forced migration increases the fear of the lack of ability of the government to control the state within the context of the current concerns regarding forced migration. In the context of this study, the forced migration theory explains the involuntary movement of the people who are internally displaced and their vulnerabilities. By implication, the phenomenon has forced many people to flee their homes, and consequently, Nigeria has become the country with the highest number of IDPs in sub-Saharan Africa, as well as living as marginal communities.

The social inclusion theory confirms the needs of the IDPs in Nigeria; the theory is centered on the group of people who requires support due to their current situation. The theory posits that in a socially inclusive society, everyone is valued, and their basic needs are supplied or provided, and by implication, the people are given a sense of belonging as reported by Robo (2014). The social inclusion theory entails the provisions of the basic needs of the people in a given society and leads to a sense of belonging among the people. Thus, IDPs required the basic necessities of life due to their susceptibility to society. According to Charity Commission (2001), social inclusion is due to the action taken sanguinely to change the circumstances of these people. In addition, everyone in the society required certain values for their survival. As observed by Robo (2014), some values form the basis of the social inclusion theory, such as everyone needs support, can learn, can contribute, can communicate, and can live together in better conditions. Thus, IDPs in the northeast require the basic values of life, such as support, care, communication, and learning, among others, for their continued existence as members of society. The social inclusive theory is appropriate for this study as it supports the integration of the IDPs into the larger society. It is observed that if IDPs are well-supported and given all the necessary care and are well-integrated into the society by implication, it can lead to better management of the plights of the IDPs and enhanced security of the nation, as well as enhanced human society and a reduction of vulnerability and marginality.

The method utilized for this study is the qualitative method, basically because of the nature of the research. The methods of data collection in this qualitative research were (1) documentary research, (2) in-depth interviews, and (3) non-participatory observation, to achieve a higher rate of response, as noted by Babbie (2013). The study took place in northeast Nigeria, which is considered one of the marginal communities as observed being the region with the highest number of IDPs and with the challenges of poor socioeconomic and health conditions. Thus, the unbearable and provoking deteriorating living conditions of the IDPs causes them to be regarded as marginal communities in sub-Saharan Africa. The selected areas of the study are the Adamawa, Borno, and Yobe states.

The sampling method utilized for this study was quota sampling, and the justification for using this method is that there is no need for callbacks and the incidence of time-wasting is equally reduced. Thus, the data were analyzed within the context of the subtopics, and the results or findings of the study were presented in a narrative form.

SOCIOECONOMIC AND HEALTH ASSESSMENT OF IDPS IN THE NORTHEAST

Living Conditions of IDPs

The living conditions of the IDPs are worrisome because of the overcrowding of the IDPs and the spread of diseases among them. The problem of overcrowding frequently arises due to the overstretched usage of the inadequate existing amenities in the camps. It is observed that the continuous influx of people into the already-congested camps makes the living conditions of the IDPs more terrible, with psychological trauma and widespread diseases as advanced by the African Centre for Strategies Studies (ACSS) (2019) and the Internal Displacement Monitoring Centre (IDMC)(2018). The continuous entry of people into these already-overcrowded camps makes the living conditions of IDPs more horrible besides the psychological trauma they experience. In addition, obtainable information revealed that endemic malaria, acute respiratory infections, and watery diarrhea are critical health concerns affecting the IDPs, with malaria featuring in 50 percent of all the health-related cases in the camps (WHO, 2018). Besides, the study found that IDPs in all the camps faced enormous challenges of leaking roofs and flooding during the rainy season. IDPs generally felt displeased and frustrated with their shelter and expressed fear over the nature of the shelter they lived in because of the danger they experienced. One of the KIs reported that:

> The Boko Haram insurgency has led to excess numbers of IDPs living in the camps with the scarcity of water and breakdown diarrhea with poor health attention, and the IDPs are still at high risk of getting communicable diseases.

Another KI revealed that:

> We are confined into a small space with congested tents with poor ventilation, and the situation is severe during the rainy period, with leakage of roofs, while mosquitos and other reptiles always have their days, and malaria, typhoid, cold, and cholera are rampant, especially among children.

The study observed that amenities, such as toilets, a steady water supply, kitchens, and electricity, were available in varied conditions in the IDP camps, but they were not sufficient to cater to all the needs of the IDPs. Hence, this study observed that BHI has contributed to the excess numbers of IDPs living in the camps with a scarcity of water, roof leakages, and widespread disease, and by implication, IDPs are at high risk of contracting communicable diseases.

Access to Education among the Children of IDPs

It is pertinent to state that this study found that there exists an alarming number of children among IDPs whose education has been truanted due to the forced displacement or death of their parents, and the breakdown of the educational system in the northeast has picked up the pace by the destruction of schools and the killing and kidnapping of pupils, students, and teachers by Boko Haram. Similarly, the study established that school facilities were provided by NGOs who have been responsible for the payment of ad-hoc staff salaries. The children were expected to join public secondary schools upon completion of their primary education within the communities. It was noticed that the learning environment is not conducive for an education due to poor instructional materials, as explained by Abdul Azeez (2016). The quality of education accessible by children of IDPs is poor and beneath the established standard because of the lack of a conducive environment for teaching and learning, as well as the absence of teaching materials. Education depends on aid and support mainly from NGOs and philanthropists for funding, provision of facilities, and teaching materials, among others. There are indications that there was no organized or logically approach to ensure the access of children to schools, and school-age children were left to the mercy of their parents with no or less formal system of the education program to ensure access to quality basic education. One of the KIs revealed that:

> The efforts of the NGOs and philanthropies are highly appreciated by building classes and providing teaching materials, but there is still the challenge of delay or nonpayment of the volunteering teachers, leading to the withdrawal of some of these teachers.

Another KI makes known that:

> The majority of the children of the IDPs are out of school, and most of the parents are poor and can hardly afford to send their children to schools, therefore, female children are married out while male children go on begging instead of going to school.

Thus, the study found that the children of the IDPs lack access to universal basic education because there is no proper arrangement for formal education, and the efforts of the NGOs and philanthropies hardly go beyond primary education. The destabilized households, as a result of forced movement of people leading to displacement, hinder the enrollment of children into schools as observed among the IDPs in northeast Nigeria. By implication, human displacement in Nigeria is equally a contributing factor to the poor or low record of enrollment of children in schools.

Crime and Drug Abuse among the IDPs

In order to get some kind of mental relief from the psychological trauma of forced displacement, many IDPs become more inclined to make use of drugs and other harmful substances, like cocaine, heroin, and marijuana, among others. The study observed that the IDPs can access these drugs from their host communities. The use of these hard drugs habitually drives victims to form gangs, which could, in due course, transform them to commit crimes as well as contribute to the spread of sexually transmitted diseases and deadly diseases, like the HIV/AIDS pandemic, through the sharing of needles during drug injections. The study found that children and women are commonly abused, due to the influence of drugs. It was reported by Olajide (2016) that there is a high occurrence of rape and other kinds of violence against women and children in IDP camps due to drug abuse. One of the KIs reported that:

> We experience cases of the use of hard drugs among adults and young people in IDPs camps. Many of the IDPs get addicted to drugs as a result of trauma from the Boko Haram insurgency, which has led to a high crime rate among IDPs.

Another KI revealed that:

> The use of drugs among the IDPs has contributed to the crime rate because there are established cases of people who engage in the use of hard drugs, misbehaving because they are out of their senses, and acting under the influence of the drugs. Even women and children abuse some of these drugs for cough.

The study established that forced displacement has led many IDPs to become drug addicts as a means of reducing tension or trauma of the displacement, and this influences their behaviour; men, women, and children are not left out of drug abuse, and by implication, they contribute to the crime rates in the society.

Livelihoods of IDPs

The study discovered that in the IDPs' camps, their livelihood activities consist of limited farming, renting motorbikes to convey passengers, and petty jobs, like cutting nails and shoe-shining. The study also found out that most of the IDPs had been farmers before their displacement, and after the forced displacement by BHI, most of the IDPs did not have access to land for cultivation. Many IDPs expressed concern over the lack of sufficient means of livelihood, with many women lamenting being redundant or idle and soliciting support to start earning a living instead of begging or relying on the government, NGOs, or philanthropies for their daily survival. This is because even when they were being taught different skills by the NGOs, they lack the capital to start a business, as revealed by one of the KIs below:

> We are tired of staying jobless or idle, but we need capital to set up a business so that we can take good care of ourselves, send our children to schools, and stop living as beggars.

Another KI revealed that:

> We were into farming activities and trading before displacement, and we were living well and taking good care of our family members. However, BHI forced us out of our homes and rendered us helpless and beggars. We relied mainly on support from the government, NGOs, and philanthropies to survive.

The study observed that before the forced displacement of the IDPs, they had different means of livelihood, such as farming and trading, among others, and their living conditions were not as bad as they are now. They were able to cater to the immediate basic needs of their family members. However, their situations are very pathetic and frustrating now, since most of them are jobless because they lost their land for cultivation and other investments due to their displacement, and the economic condition of the country is not stable, which has resulted in how they survive now at the mercy of support from the government, NGOs, and philanthropies. Hence, the lack of adequate means of livelihood forms a major challenge for the IDPs and contributes to the high rate of unemployment of the people of the northeast. As explained by Ejiofor, Oni, and Sejoro (2017), the unemployment rate in the northeast stood at 60 percent, which is on the high side.

Poverty and Hunger

The blight of poverty can be noticed across Nigeria, as evidenced by the standard of living of the majority in the country. The study observed the low household income that traverses the country and poor economic instability, which further makes complex the wretchedness of the IDPs. The study found that the bulk of IDPs in the camps are only getting measly rations of food that can hardly fulfill their nutritional needs as required for the human body. Hence, as a result of hunger, the nutritional intakes, particularly among the children in these camps, are very poor, leading to high mortality and morbidity of children, especially those under the age of five. The women and the aged form the largest group of the IDPs who are severely affected. Thus, IDPs are facing a severe food shortage, insecurity, and living under severe poverty and hunger, as noted by one of the KIs below:

> The circumstances regarding feeding are pitiable and regrettable as we hardly get enough food to cater to our nutritional needs. We are living in hunger and abject poverty, and our children are malnourished with hunger-related diseases. We can hardly cater to our family members due to poverty and hunger.

Another KI disclosed that:

> We are hungry because we are poor and living under abject poverty and hunger due to forced displacement. Life was good for us before the insurgency and living in the IDP camps. Feeding was good and regular at the early stage of the camps, but reduced gradually, and the quality of the food is generally poor while the majority of the IDPs depend on food from NGOs and philanthropies.

Therefore, this study observed that the IDPs are living in hunger and poverty, and food continues to be a major requirement, as most of the IDPs continue to barter for themselves with little support from NGOs and philanthropies. Some of the IDPs (men, women, and children) engage in menial or seasonal jobs available in their areas to support their family members. The study further observed that the IDPs are not happy with the feeding systems while living in hunger and poverty, because the menial jobs they are doing can hardly cater to the immediate needs of their family members. This contributes to the lowest human development index, as elucidated by Onaedo, Samuel, and Sejoro (2017). The north is known to have the lowest human development index in Nigeria, with 71.5 percent of northeasterners living below the internationally recognized poverty line. In addition, IDPs suffer low-nutritional-value food. As observed by Dunn (2018), IDPs are facing severe food insecurity and nutritional problems with a global acute malnutrition level of 27.3 percent.

Poor Environment Maintenance and Water Contamination

The study found that one of the main risk factors associated with the increase of infectious diseases is poor environmental management, water pollution, overstretched usage of the inadequate accessible amenities in these camps, and the additional trooping of people into these camps. This makes the situations of IDPs worse, and by implication, it affects the health of the IDPs. In Nigeria, there are established cases of many environmentally hazardous practices like open defecation and poor household disposals. The study further observes the high practice of open defecation and other environmental degradation in IDP camps. The passing of these solid wastes frequently makes its way back to water sources present in these camps, which most of them equally find useful for drinking and use for other domestic activities.

This poor sanitation depicts a high risk to the public health of IDPs and serves as a source of ill-health conditions, consequently endangering the lives of IDPs and aiding in the spread of diseases. It is noted from the obtainable information revealed that endemic malaria, typhoid, and watery diarrhea are critical health-alarming diseases affecting the IDPs as a result of poor water and sanitation facilities. It was reported by one of the KIs that:

> The shortage of water and toilet facilities makes the majority of the IDPs practice open defecation, and this has led to breakdown and diarrhea with poor health attention and IDPs are at high risk of getting communicable diseases.

Another KI revealed that:

> We the IDPs noticed that poor environmental management and water pollution contributes mainly to the spread of contagious disease, especially among children and aged people.

Consequently, the study found that one of the major risk factors for the spread of many infectious diseases is poor environmental management and water pollution. The absence of waste management and inadequate provision of essential utilities such as potable water and good sanitary conditions has led to poor sanitation and hygiene, and by implication it causes the frequent outbreak of diseases like cholera and other related illnesses. As reported by the United Nations Children's Emergency Fund (UNICEF, 2016), with the trooping of IDPs into the camps, the available water and sanitation facilities and structure became inadequate to accommodate the essential needs of the IDPs, which eventually increases the risk of the spread of diseases, dehydration, and other related ailments.

Health Care of IDPs

The study discovered that BHI has undermined the global health quality services because the IDPs lack access to quality health-care services, as most of the medical facilities have been attacked and closed down. Most of the clinics in these IDP camps were constructed by NGOs and philanthropies with few medical personnel. The IDPs collectively agreed that access to health services is a major concern, because there is no logical and efficient health management to cater to the health needs of the IDPs, and women, especially pregnant women and children, as well as the aged, suffer more. The study further observed that the health conditions of the IDPs became worse due to unemployment and poverty, as well as their inability to cater to their medical needs. Thus, the IDPs hardly get basic health-care services, and BHI attacks that led to forced displacement have become threats to public health and affect the safe delivery of universal quality health service to conflict, depressing IDPs, as revealed by KIs below:

> Forced displacement because of the Boko Haram Insurgency makes it difficult for the IDPs to get appropriate health attention, because there are many of us having a serious illness that needs medical checkups always, but there is a shortage of medical personnel, medical facilities, and drugs.

Another KI stressed that:

> Boko Haram attacks put off regular access to quality health service with shortage of drugs and most of the health personnel are always afraid to stay in the camps to attend to IDPs.

Consequently, IDPs have the challenges of access to health care, water, sanitation, and hygiene, as well as theft. As observed by Global Overview (GO) (2015), the Boko Haram insurgency fighters have attacked many health facilities and health workers, leaving IDPs with poor access to health care, sanitation, and hygiene. Hence, it is observed that frequent Boko Haram insurgency attacks that led to forced displacement have affected quality health services, and by implication, access to universal quality health services has become unachievable and by inference has worsened the health conditions of IDPs. To this end, repeated threats to public service providers by insurgents and the overpopulation of the IDPs, with limited health personnel and facilities, affect the delivery of quality health services to violence distressed IDPs.

To this end, Ngige, Badekale, and Hammanjoda (2016) expressed that globally insurgency has despondently become one of the recounting features of our society today. It is worth noting that Nigeria as a country is not left out of the affliction of IDPs. As observed by Heerten and Moses (2017), Nigeria, like other nations in the worried sub-Sahara Africa, is not free from the afflictions of IDPs. It is observed that BHI flourish in northern Nigeria due to the poor socioeconomic conditions of the people. As advanced by Oyewole (2017), the socioeconomic authenticity of northern Nigeria is rooted in the colonial period with corruption and poor governance that produced a favourable environment for various dissident movements that employ religious prejudice and intolerance to gain legitimacy.

Boko Haram has desolately become one of the defining features of northeast Nigeria and as a thought connected openly to the global web of fundamental Islamists' philosophy and the doctrines of Boko Haram linked to Muhammad Yusuf based on the principles of rejecting conventional education, disapproval of secularism and Westernization, and the inaptness of Islam with democracy (Raineri & Martini, 2017). Thus, Boko Haram launched a series of attacks on public places and citizens and radiated misgivings in the minds of citizens of the government's failure to secure them, making them feel unprotected and vulnerable has resulted in the flow of thousands of people into internally displaced persons camps seeking shelter, protection, and other support, thus, becoming marginal communities in sub-Saharan Africa.

It is also important to note that all these states where the IDPs look for shelter, security, and other supports are also affected by the BHI, which led to a struggle over the insufficient resources between the IDPs and the host communities (Eweka & Olusegun, 2016; National Emergency Management Agency [NEMA], 2016). Thus, BHI has led to serious competition over the limited resources between the host communities and IDPs, and by implication, they led to another form of tragedy. Thus, it is observed that IDPs experience poor living conditions and are faced with many challenges, ranging from poor government policies, sexual abuse, poor shelter, and a lack of food, as well as the absence of quality health services, and by implication, undermining the reintegration of IDPs into the communities and gaining a long-lasting way out of the challenges facing the IDPs. Therefore, it can be deduced that BHI created an unbearable challenge for IDPs, thus provoking the deteriorating living conditions of IDPs despite the effort put in place by the government and other stakeholders to improve the socioeconomic and health conditions of the IDPs, who are observed as one of the marginal communities in sub-Saharan Africa.

DISCUSSIONS AND CONCLUSION

The study discovered that the effects of IDPs on any given society are immense, and as such, the instability and wretchedness, as well as loss of lives, affect the economy and threaten the health of the human population. BHI has led to a huge loss of lives and the breakdown of the family structure and the destruction of property. The study observed that the displacement of individuals as a result of natural disasters or insurgencies like Boko Haram has led to the dysfunction of the socioeconomic and health systems of society. The IDPs lose their valuables, homes, and places of work, businesses, household income, and other forms of investments. In addition, public facilities that have scarce resources are destroyed, making life more difficult for IDPs. In addition, the displacement of people not only affects the IDPs' household income, but it has crippled every socioeconomic and health structure of society by paralyzing the supply chain. Both internal and external business investors, like financial institutions, telecommunication companies, schools, and hospitals, among others, in the insurgency-prone areas stand at risk of poor financial performance and job cuts, and by implication they are seen as marginal communities in sub-Saharan Africa.

The study found that many IDPs are at risk of poverty, hunger, and disease, as well as living as marginal communities in sub-Saharan Africa, and these assertions agreed with the work of IDMC (2018) that globally, the displacement of people from their places of domicile has become a recurring problem with social, health, and economic burden. Similarly, IDPs are faced with challenges of poor accessibility to food, nutrition, health care, shelter, water, sanitation, and education, among others, and they corroborate the assertion of UNOCHA (2018) that IDPs in northeast Nigeria are in serious need of life-saving support, such as food and nutrition, health care, shelter, and non-food items, potable water, and improved sanitation and hygiene conditions.

It is also vital to state that most of the burden of the forced IDPs happened in the developing countries, with children worse affected. As noted by UNHCR (2017), about 85 percent of the burden of forced displaced people transpires among the developing nations of the world, and 52 percent of the incidences are among children below eighteen years of age and by implication they are regarded as marginal communities in sub-Saharan Africa. Thus, it is observed that women and children form the highest number of IDPs who experience serious neglect, and they are faced with many challenges ranging from poor government policies, sexual abuse, poor shelter, and food, as well as the absence of quality health services, and by implication, undermining their reintegration IDPs into the communities and getting long-lasting way out of the challenges facing the IDPs and implication living in deteriorating conditions as marginal communities in sub-Saharan Africa. Hence, it is pertinent to point out that the number of IDPs in different IDP camps and other host communities remains a major national burden in Nigeria with socioeconomic and health consequences and as marginal communities in Africa.

Thus, this chapter concludes with the fact that insurgencies are considered one of the main barriers to social, political, and quality health services globally, and by implication, IDPs are considered to be marginal communities, and concerted efforts through legal and political channels are required to address the challenges of growing conflicts and insurgencies in northeast Nigeria. Socioeconomic stability and quality health services will become unattainable, especially for IDPs, who are victims of insurgencies, and they also vulnerable to poor quality service and implications. These continue to lower Nigeria's ranking in global socioeconomic and health indicators and as marginal communities in sub-Saharan Africa.

From the study presented in this chapter, it is imperative to ensure improved socioeconomic and health situations of IDPs as a marginalized community in northeast Nigeria. To achieve this, government has to guarantee strong national socioeconomic and health policies and strategies in line with world best practices. The Nigerian government needs to make possible a peace process that can restrict the insurgency activities in northeast Nigeria. There is a need to upgrade the existing IDP camps to make them fit for human habitation. The government needs to strengthen the existing relationship with national and international NGOs as well as philanthropies, especially in the areas of socioeconomic empowerment and health of the IDPs. The government also needs to guarantee that aid given for the well-being of IDPs are well-utilized and documented, made accountable for, and prevent any form of diversion. The resettlement of IDPs needs to be taken more seriously, with the main concern being the rebuilding process to hasten the safe return of the IDPs.

NOTE

The researcher conducted this study in compliance with ethical requirements. Informed consent was observed. During the interviews, the respondents were secured and unharmed. All the respondents were anonymized and granted their confidentiality with respect to their privacy.

ACKNOWLEDGMENT

The researcher would also like to thank all the key informants who provided useful information for this research.

REFERENCES

Abdul Azeez, M. (2016). The Boko Haram Insurgency and Internal Displacement. State Secretariat for Migration. SEM. Retrieved October 2, 2018, from https://www.sem.admin.ch/dam/data/sem/internationals/harkumftslaender/afrika/nga-boko.haram.e.pdf.

Africa Centre for Strategies Studies [ACSS]. (2019). Population Displacement in Africa: Top 10 Countries of Origin. Retrieved May 2, 2020, from https://africacenter.org/spotlight/population-displacement-africa.

Asplet, M. (2013). Internal Displacement: Responsibility and Action. Retrieved October 2, 2020 from http://archive.ipu.org/PDF/publications/Displacement-e.pdf.

Babbie, E. (2013). *The Practice of Social Research*. 19th ed. Wadsworth. Cengage Learning.

Bhagwan, K.S. (2013). Conflict-Driven Internal Persons in Manipur: Legal and Human Security Framework. Master's Dissertation, Sikkim University, Gangtok.

Benz, S., and Hasenclever, A. (2009). *The Global Governance of Forced Migration.* Paper Presented at the ECPR Joint Session 2009 14–19 April, Libson Portugai (Workshop No. 27) University of Tubingen/Germany.

Castles, S. (2009). Development and Migration or Migration and Development. What Comes First? *Asian and Pacific Migration Journal*, 18(4): 441–71.

Displacement Tracking Matrix. (2017). Displacement Tracking Matrix: Nigeria Round XV Report 2017. Retrieved from https://data2.unhcr.org/en/documents/download/56254.

Dunn, G. (2018). The Impact of the Boko Haram Insurgency in Northeast Nigeria on Childhood Wasting a Double Difference Study, *Conflict and Health*, 12(1): 6.

Ejiofor, O.C., Oni, S., and Sejoro, J.V. (2017). An Assessment of the Impact of Internal Displacement of Human Security in Northern Nigeria. *Acta Universitatis*, 10(1): 19–42.

Eweka, O., and Olesegun, T.O. (2016). Management of Internally Displaced Persons in Africa: Comparing Nigeria and Cameroon. *African Research Review*, 10(1): 6.

Ezra, G., Ekundayo, A., and Samson, B.A. (2014). Possible Determinants and Spatial Patterns of Anaemia among Young Children in Nigeria: A Bayesian Semi-Parametric Modelling. Retrieved March 3, 2018 from https://www.researchgate.net/publication/260023562_Possible_determinants_and_spatial_patterns_of_anaemia_among_young_children_in_Nigeria_a_Bayesian_semi_parametric_modelling.

Fouka, G., and Mantzorou, M. (2011). What Are the Major Ethical Issues in Conducting Research? Is There a Conflict between the Research Ethics and the Nature of Nursing? *Health Science Journal,* 5(1): 3–14.

Global Overview (GO). (2015). People Internally Displaced by Conflict and Violence. *International Displacement Monitoring Committee (IDMC)*: 8–64.

Heerten, I., and Moses, A.D. (2017). *Post-Colonial Conflict and the Questions of Genocide Routledge*. Retrieved April 10, 2018 from https://doi.org/10.432/97813152229294.

Internal Displacement Monitoring Centre [IDMC]. (2018). The Ripple Effect: Economic Impacts of Internal Displacement. Retrieved July 2, 2020, from http://www.internal-displacement.org/sites/default/files/inline-files/-idmc-economic-impacts-intro-0.pdf.

Kevin, M. D. (2018). Forced Migration and Displacement in Africa: Contexts, Causes and Consequences, *African Geographical Review,* 37(2): 79–82.

National Emergency Management in Nigeria (NEMA). (2016). Borno Still Has 32 IDP Camps Despite Returns of Some Displaced Persons. Abuja: NEMA.

Ngige, C.V., Badekale, A.F., and Hammanjoda, I. (2016). The Media and Boko Haram Insurgency in Nigeria: A Content Analysis and Review. *International Journal of Peace and Conflict Studies*, 3(1): 58–65.

Norwegian Refugee Council [NRC]. (2017). New Study: Displaced Nigerians too Scared to Return Home. Retrieved October 2, 2018, from https://www.nre.no.news/2017/october-displaced-nigerians-too-scared-to-return-home.

Olajide, A. (2016). Investigation: How Nigerian Women and Children Fare in IDPs Camps (Parts 1). Retrieved October 2, 2018, from https//politics.naij.com/812953-Investigation-Nigerian-women-children-fare-idps-camps-part-1-html.

Onaedo, E., Samuel, O., and Sejoro, J. (2017). An Assessment of the Impact of Internal Displacement on Human Security in Northern Nigeria. *Acta Universitatis Danubius Relations Internationales*, 10(1): 42–65.

Oyewole, S. (2017). Making the Sky Relevant to Battle Strategy: Counterinsurgency and the Prospects of Air Power in Nigeria. *Studies in Conflict & Terrorism*, *40*(3): 211–31. https://doi.org/10.1080/1057610X.2016.1188533.

Raineri, L., and Martini, A. (2017). ISIS and Al-Qaeda as Strategies and Political Imaginaries in Africa: A Comparison between Boko Haram and Al-Qaeda in the Islamic Maghreb. *Civil Wars*, 19(4): 425–47. https://doi org/10.1080/13698249.20117.1413226.

Robo, M. (2014). Social Inclusion and Inclusive Education. *Academicus International Scientific Journal.* Retrieved November 21, 2018, from http://www.academicus.edu.al/nr10/Academicus-MMXIV-10-181-191.pdf.

The Charity Commission. (2001). *The Promotion of Social Inclusion*. Design, Charity Commission. Retrieved September 23, 2010 from www.charitycommission.gov.uk.

Umar, S.S., Suleiman, M.S., and Magaji, R.A. (2018). Assessment of Health Risks among Vulnerable Groups of Internally Displaced Persons in Pompomari Camp, Damaturu, Yobe State, Nigeria. *IGWEBUIKE: An African Journal of Arts and Humanities.*

United Nations Children's Emergency Fund [UNICEF]. (2016). UNICEF Nigeria—Water, Sanitation, and Hygiene—Providing Lifesaving Interventions in Water, Sanitation and Hygiene for Internally Displaced Persons in Northeast Nigeria. Retrieved May 7, 2018, from https://www.unicef.org/nigeria/wes 10558html.

United Nations Refugee Agency [UNHCR]. (2017). Global Trend in Forced Displacement in 2017. Retrieved October 2, 2020, from https://www.unhcr.org/globaltrends.

United Nations Office for the Coordination of Humanitarian Affairs [UNOCHA]. (2018). About OCHA Nigeria | OCHA. Retrieved April 6, 2018, from http:www.unocha.org/nigeria/about-ocha-nigeria.

United Nations-Habitat. (2018). *The Right to Adequate Housing*. Fact Sheet No. 21/Rev.1 Retrieved July 7, 2021, from https://www.ohchr.org/Documents/Publications/FS21_rev_ 1-Housing_en.pdf.

World Health Organization [WHO]. (2018). Malaria Campaign Saving Young Lives in Nigeria. Retrieved June 5, 2020, from http://www.who.int/malaria/news/emergency-borno-state/en/.

Chapter 12

Intergenerational Patterns of Adolescent Sexual Activities

The Impact of the Nigerian Civil War in Abia State, Nigeria

Chigozirim Ogubuike, Olukemi K. Amodu, and Mofeyisara Oluwatoyin Omobowale

INTRODUCTION

The World Health Organization (WHO) defines *adolescents* as individuals between ten and nineteen years of age (WHO, 2015). Adolescence is a critical developmental period and is understood as the years between the onset of puberty and the establishment of social independence (Steinberg, 2014). The most readily recognized hallmark of adolescence is the pubertal metamorphosis, orchestrating the visible transformation of a "child" into an "adult" (Curtis, 2015). During adolescence, there is physical, psychological, and emotional development triggered by a cascade of endocrine changes that lead to sexual maturation and reproductive capability (UN, 2012; UNICEF, 2012). As adolescents attain puberty, there is an earnest search for friendship, intimacy, and relationship opportunities, which makes them susceptible to sexual activity. We focused on adolescents' sexual activities in the traditional Igbo society over time, from the pre-civil war period to contemporary times.

In traditional Igbo society, sex was rarely discussed. It was considered sacrilegious for adults to discuss sexuality-related matters either with or in the presence of the young. It was also inappropriate for adolescents to discuss sex with their elders (Onuche, 2014). The girls were required to be very pure and moral, with a focus on their virginity. Because a female child is sexually more susceptible than a male child, because she can become pregnant, but a guy cannot, the moral judgment was aimed primarily at female children (Amadiume, 2005). Any girl who loses her virginity before marriage is viewed as a dishonour to her parents and a disappointment to the husband (Agbogu & Igbokwe, 2015), but a virgin bride draws many presents and goodwill. Sexual freedom outside of marriage was not permitted and remains a source of shame, particularly for mothers who were traditionally expected to assist their adolescent daughters in giving their husbands their most valuable asset—their virginity (Uche, 2009). Adolescents who are caught engaging in sexual activity are mocked through songs, lyrics, and folktales, and the parents of these children are publicly humiliated and judged as failures (Onwuama & Adepoju, 2010). The patterns of adolescent sexual behaviour in Igbo society are, nevertheless, evolving.

Environmental influences have a significant impact on a child's behaviour, according to Bronfenbrenner's ecological systems theory. This environmental component includes environmental events, life-course transitions, socio-historical circumstances, and cultural changes (Bronfenbrenner, 1979). According to John (2018), culture change is the gradual alteration of a group's shared way of life. These changes may be sudden or gradual. A situation that abruptly altered culture and had an impact on adolescents' health and behavior was the Nigerian civil war. According to the ecological systems theory, in the chrono-system layer when there are environmental events that lead to transitions over the life course, it may exert a direct or indirect influence on other ecological system layers. The Nigerian civil war was a notable environmental event that had caused a culture change over time affecting the family, health, and sexual activities. This event influenced the attitudes and cultural ideologies in the Igbo society.

The Nigerian civil war was fought between eastern Nigeria, known during the war as "Biafra," and the federal government of Nigeria, from July 6, 1967, to January 12, 1970. It was the first modern war in post-independence sub-Saharan Africa, fought in the southeastern region, and it resulted in the deaths of between one and three million people (Akresh et al., 2012; Akresh et al., 2017). During the war, many men died, leaving their wives defenceless. Children were more vulnerable to sex, and prostitution was viewed as a way to survive (Akresh et al., 2017). Girls were increasingly being sexually exploited and raped by both Nigerian and Biafran soldiers during the conflict (Smith, 2005). According to reports, parents were exchanging their girls for food and security (Akresh et al., 2017). The town was also put in danger during the conflict because some of the Nigerian soldiers raped and fled with women, who worked as spies, sex workers, and "army wives." When the "army wives" returned to the community after the war, it led to friction, since some of the "army wives" brought along children whose army fathers had deserted them. Premarital pregnancies, youth internal elopement, and the exploitation of certain sexual rites and rituals all began at this time (Nwashindu & Ihediwa, 2016).

Researchers have reported findings from contemporary adolescent sexual activities in Igbo society (Smith, 2000; Smith, 2005; Onwubiko et al., 2015). Communities in Abia state were marginalised as a result of the Nigerian civil war, making it one of the affected states in the southeastern region. In order to examine premarital sexuality as a sign and result of changes connected with "modernity" in Igboland, a school-based study was undertaken in Umuahia, the capital of Abia state, among students aged fourteen to twenty-one. It found that roughly 36 percent of the students had engaged in sexual activity. Boys were more likely than girls to report having sex, with 48.1 percent of boys and 27.7 percent of girls reporting having sex, respectively (Smith, 2000). More than 70 percent of Igbo-speaking adolescents and young adults in Aba and Kano who were between the ages of fifteen and twenty-four reported engaging in sexual activity, with slightly more females than men having such experiences in Aba (71 percent versus 67 percent), according to a qualitative study (Smith, 2005). In Aba, a school-based study conducted among secondary school students found that 18 percent of the adolescents were sexually active (Onwubiko et al., 2015).

Adolescents' involvement in sexual activities exposes them to deleterious outcomes, which include experiencing sexually transmitted infections (STIs), including HIV, unplanned pregnancies, and unsafe abortions. Nigeria has the second-highest number of people living with HIV/AIDs worldwide (NDHS, 2013; UNAIDS, 2018). More than two million adolescents aged ten to nineteen years old are living with HIV. About one in seven of all new HIV infections occur during adolescence (UNFPA, 2015). HIV prevalence among adolescent girls aged fifteen to nineteen years is far too high, and a large proportion of the new infections occur among adolescent girls (UNAIDs, 2014). Adolescents who have HIV are subjected to stigma, discrimination, and human rights violations, all of which have a detrimental effect on their general well-being. A significant factor in maternal and infant mortality, as well as intergenerational cycles of illness and poverty, is adolescent pregnancy (WHO, 2018). Adolescent pregnancy has a variety of social repercussions, from ostracism, where advantages are taken away from the unwed mothers, to threats of violence, poor education, school dropout rates, the breeding of social miscreants, and poverty (Adetoro, 2010; Ayuba and Gani, 2012; Olurinola, 2016; WHO, 2018). Every year, females between fifteen and nineteen years old have over 3.9 million unsafe abortions, which contribute to maternal deaths and long-term health issues (Darroch, 2016).

Studies have been conducted on adolescent sexual behaviours and practises (Nwankwo and Nwoke, 2009; Duru et al., 2010; Azuike et al., 2015; Nlewem and Amodu, 2017). However, intergenerational patterns of adolescent sexual activities are understudied. It is, therefore, imperative to interrogate intergenerational patterns of sexual activities among adolescents in Abia state and explain the possible contribution of an environmental event (the Nigerian civil war) to the observed patterns in the selected marginalised communities in Abia state.

MATERIALS AND METHODS

Study Area

Abia state is one of Nigeria's thirty-six states located in the southeastern region of Nigeria. It has a population census of about 4,112,230, with a density of 650/km2 (Federal Republic of Nigeria official *Gazette*, 2007). Abia state is divided into seventeen LGAs and is bordered on the north and northeast by the states of Anambra, Enugu, and Ebonyi. The state capital is Umuahia, while Aba is the largest city and commercial centre. After achieving independence in 1960, Abia state was part of the post-independence Eastern Region until 1967, when the region was split and the area became part of the East Central state. After about two months, the former Eastern Region attempted to secede (causing the Nigerian civil war), with Abia as a part of the secessionist state of Biafra. As the war ended, the East Central state was reformed, and in 1976, Imo state (including Abia) was formed by the Murtala Muhammed regime. After about fifteen years, the eastern Imo state was divided to form Abia state in 1991. The contemporary Abia state has been inhabited for years by various ethnic groups, primarily the Igbo people (Hoiberg, 2010).

Study Design, Population, Sample Size Estimation, and Sampling Technique

A cross-sectional study design was conducted using a qualitative approach to explore intergenerational patterns of adolescent sexual activities. The study was carried out in four randomly selected local government areas in Abia state, namely Aba North, Aba South, Osisioma, and Obioma Ngwa local governments influenced by the war.

The study populations were adolescents at different timeframes, spanning the period of 1957 to 2019. The age group of the study participants from the different eras includes pre–civil war (seventy-one to eighty years); civil war time (sixty-one to seventy years); post–civil war (fifty-one to sixty years); and contemporary adolescents (ten to nineteen years). The participants who were included in the study were individuals who fell into the age brackets for each era and had experiences of the study phenomena. Those who consented to participate in the study were also included. Participants excluded from this study were individuals with memory loss, those who were ill at the time of the study, and those who were not indigenes of the LGA and state of study.

Thirty respondents participated in this study (eight participated in a life-history interview while twenty-two participated in an in-depth interview). Both snowballing and purposive sampling techniques were used in recruiting participants for this study. Snowballing sampling techniques were used in recruiting individuals into the life-history interviews, and purposive sampling was used in recruiting participants into the in-depth interviews.

Data Collection Methods/Instrument/Procedure

The data collection methods used in the study were archival research, life-history interviews, and in-depth interviews. An archival checklist was used to search and review materials from the archives. Information on adolescent sexual activities and civil war experiences were elicited from intelligent reports, newspapers, books, bulletins, and all other relevant documents from the National Archives in Enugu and Ibadan. The archival research method was conducted first before proceeding with the other data-collection methods. The guides were developed based on reviews of the literature. Prior to the commencement of data collection, community entry was conducted in the local government area of study, and permission was sought from the community development chairman (CDC) and the council of chiefs. The purpose of the study was explained to the participants, and those who consented to participate in the study gave both written and verbal informed consent.

Data Analysis and Management

Recorded interviews were transcribed immediately after the interviews to guarantee completeness that could be lost by delay. Transcription was verbatim, as this process protects the originality and reliability of the data collected. The interviews conducted in Igbo were translated and transcribed into English. The typed transcripts were read several times and cleaned; the transcripts were coded; and a code book was developed both inductively and deductively with themes, subthemes, and codes. Data was analysed using the thematic analysis method with Atlas data qualitative software version 7.5.21. A clear, coherent, and integrated presentation of data was done in a sequential manner.

Ethical Considerations

Before the onset of data collection, ethical approval to conduct the study was obtained from the UI/UCH Ethical Review Board and Abia state ethical review board. The participants who agreed to participate in the interviews were given a written consent form to sign after the study had been explained to them. The recorded interviews were kept private and made only available to the research teams for transcription, and the interviews were kept private and safe. Participation in the study was purely voluntary.

FINDINGS

Intergenerational Patterns of Adolescent Sexual Activities

The historical patterns of adolescent sexuality were explored and compared with contemporary times (from the colonial era, 1901–1959; pre–civil war, 1960–1966; civil war time, 1967–1970; post–civil war, 1971–1980; and contemporary times, 1990–current time). The themes explored were early marriage and betrothal, sexual initiations, sexual practice, transactional sex, and sexual communications.

Colonial Era (1901–1959): Early Marriage and Betrothal

Early marriages and betrothals were common during the colonial era. Families betrothed their children as soon as they were born. This early betrothal was reported to accompany the exchange of material gifts and favor. It was stated that after that, the girl would undergo female genital mutilation (cutting). An archival report noted that:

> Families were in the habit of betrothing infants to adults and often infants as early as the first day of birth by the exchange of symbolic gifts or rites. At the point of the exchange of this gift, the girl's clitoris will be cut if it was not done when she was an infant. (District office 1922, CSE 36/1/1)

After betrothal, the girl is engaged to the boy, and in some situations, the girl is expected to reside with the boy's family, where her character and personality are observed. This process produced familiarization between the families. Another archival dataset stated that:

> Connection with an unmarried girl who owing to the custom of early betrothal must invariably be engaged (Talbot 1926, NHB/C/4).

The girl betrothed had no choice but to accept the spouse to whom she was betrothed, or she faced the risk of being sold into slavery. Another source reported that:

> Formerly, in the case of an infant marriage, the girl, as reaching marriageable age, had no choice but to comply according to choice, and she was liable to be sold to slavery if she obstinately refused to follow the suitor selected for her by her parents. (District office 1922, CSE 36/1/1)

Other girls who were not betrothed remained in their parents' house until adolescence, when they came of marriageable age. At this point, they would receive a mark before marriage. In a way, this process of receiving marks and marriage may help in maintaining sexual purity among female adolescents, because if a girl gets pregnant before then, the marriage is postponed. According to Thomas:

> In the process of marriage where the suitor is accepted, the girl receives "*mbubu marks*" down her chest, and then the girl goes to the fattening room, *mpu,* for four months. If the girl conceives, the marking is postponed, and it is impossible for her to be marked. But if the girl does not conceive, she comes out on Afo day and the next day goes to her husband's house in the afternoon, accompanied by the mother and others. (Thomas [1913], A1/T74)

In the colonial era, adolescent boys share accommodations with the other children of the family until they attain puberty, when they are made to relocate to a separate quarter—"bachelor apartment"—and they were free to entertain special friends. These separate living arrangements may predispose them to early sexual initiation. This was vivid in Basden's report:

> A lady shares the house accommodation with the other children of the family until the age of puberty. At this stage in his life, he is allotted separate quarters, which his father may provide, but which he more likely has to build for himself. It is a tiny bachelor apartment, where he sleeps, stores his treasure, and receives his "special friends." (Basden [1921], A1/B2)

It was also revealed that love was not associated with native relationships. It was reported that when a boy meets a girl who attracts his emotions, he immediately inquires about her parents and learns her engagement status.

Sexual Initiation

Early sexual initiation is allegedly reported to occur as soon as adolescents attain puberty. An archival source averred that:

> Young women and male adolescents will indulge in sexual intercourse as soon as they attain the age of puberty. (District office 1922, CSE 36/1/10)

This is because at attaining puberty, the girl will undergo fattening at the expense of the husband-to-be in her father's compound. It was reported that:

> On the attainment of the age of puberty, the girl will be fattened at the expense of the bridegroom in her father's compound. (District office 1922, CSE 36/1/1)

During the fattening process, the girl was not allowed to do anything; she was constantly supplied with food and entertained friends. This was termed the most enjoyable part of the girls' lives. She receives care and gifts, especially from her betrothed. Another archival source averred that:

> She is not allowed to do anything and is only supplied with food and entertained by friends. It is the most enjoyable part of the girls' lives. She receives care and presents, especially from her betrothed. (Talbolt (1926), NHB/C/4)

Sexual Practice/Sexual License

In the colonial era, a sexual relationship was accepted in the concept of "sexual license." This is a situation in which the mother of the adolescent girl gives consent to the boyfriend, who seeks sexual intimacy with the daughter after a monetary offer. This was vivid, as reported by Thomas:

> Normally, a girl begins her sexual life with a boy of 15 to 16 years, who takes two shillings to her mother and says he wants to be friends with her. In the morning, the boy gives four yams to the girl. When she conceives, which they are usually careful to avoid doing till they have received their body marks, the girl goes to her husband and the boy looks out for another friend. (Thomas [1913], A1/T74)

Adolescent girls begin to have sex after they might have been betrothed to a man for marriage; they select their friends and become intimate with them. This is averred in the archival material that:

> Among young people, morals are not very rigid, the only real stipulation being that a girl must have no intimate relations with any other man prior to the first visit to her intended husband. After that is over, she is more or less free to select her own friends and invariably does so. "Should a child be born in the waiting time before actual marriage, it is the property of her betrothed husband." (Basden [1921], A1/B2)

Transactional Sex

In the colonial era, adolescent girls were used to entertain male guests. In this practice, the girls had no say, and no form of contraceptives was used by either party. The girl is not allowed to get married, but she would reside in her father's house. This was revealed in archival records, as shown in the quotes below.

One or more daughters are retained at home for life. They are kept at home solely for the entertainment of guests. Her face is tattooed with peculiar 'ichi' marks, and she is not allowed to marry, nor to reside anywhere but at her father's house. Children born from the various liaisons between her and her father's guests become part of her father's household (Basden, 1921, A1/B2).

Adolescent girls were presented as gifts to earn favor from those in authority, thus promoting promiscuous sexual behavior and increasing their risk of contracting sexually transmitted infections. Basden also reported that:

> Girls were presented by their guardians to men who occupied positions of authority in order to win favour or assistance in some business—legal or otherwise. They are offered and accepted as gifts, with the donors expecting to receive certain wives' benefits in exchange in lieu of money. (Basden [1921], A1/B2)

Sexual Communication

Adolescent girls appeared naked as part of the Ibo culture of dressing. This may in turn enhance sexual intimacy with the opposite sex and indirect sexual communication. The quotes below illustrate that:

> "It is the custom for girls to go entirely naked up to (and sometimes after) marriage." On reaching the age of puberty, a piece of fine cotton string is worn loosely around the loins to indicate the fact, and this is later discarded for a more permanent circlet of spring-coiled brass wire (called awna-idide, i.e., brass worm). (Basden [1921], A1/B2)

Much attention was paid to female hairdressing, especially during the onset of puberty, because the hair possessed great powers of attraction for the opposite sex. This may also be a form of sexual communication. This was reported that:

> The hair itself signifies much, and great pains are taken to secure a flourishing growth, as it is reckoned to possess great powers of attraction for the opposite sex. Until the age of self-consciousness and personal vanity is reached, the hair receives but scanty attention, but between this age and until a few years after

> marriage, many Ibo women exercise all their arts and spend much later time on hair dressing. (Basden [1921], A1/B2)

PRE–CIVIL WAR (1960–1966)

Early Marriage and Betrothal

Early marriages were reported in the colonial era and pre–civil war times. It was reported that parents betrothed their daughters from childhood, and the girl went to the husband's house during adolescence. This was expressed in the following quotes:

> In those days, our parents gave away girls in marriage right from when they were babies. Early marriages were common. (Aba North_Male Key Informant_78 years)

Another participant reported that:

> Generally, marrying early was common. I was married at 10 years old to a man I didn't know, and I had no choice. By 15 years, the man came to pay my bride price. (Osisioma_Female Key Informant_72 years)

Sexual Initiations

In the colonial era, early sexual initiations were revealed, especially during puberty and after going for fattening. Prior to the war, it was revealed that sexual freedom was repressed after the colonial era (1960).

It was reported that the premarital chastity of an adolescent was very important to the mother, and she would do anything within her power to ensure the girl kept it. This was vivid in archival material:

> A mother's reputation was deeply involved in her daughter's pre-marital chastity, and she would do everything possible to preserve it and avoid a scandal. (Ifemesia [1979], NHB/C/93)

It was further narrated that in the end, if the girl maintained her virginity, the mother would be publicly congratulated:

> In the end, on the daughter's marriage, the mother would be publicly congratulated and munificently rewarded by an appreciative son-in-law. (Ifemesia [1979], NHB/C/93)

In-depth interviews also revealed that sex wasn't a regular thing in pre–civil war times. It was revealed that their minds weren't on initiating sexual intercourse because most of them were preoccupied with farmwork. The quotes below buttress some of the claims:

> It wasn't a regular thing. You can't tell a girl to come, let's go and have sex. It means you are a devil . . . Then before a girl will say, "That's my boyfriend." It is always very hard for a boy to say. (Aba North_Male respondent_78 years)

Another participant further revealed that:

> Things were better then. Young boys and girls could freely be naked and work around the community. If sex was not too common, then our minds were not fixed on those things then. We may have seen naked ladies, but our minds were not there for sex. If it was now, there would have been a problem. Our minds were on going to the farm and helping out with farmwork. (Obingwa_Male respondent_74 years)

It was further explained by one of the female respondents that expressing sexual feelings by the man wasn't as easy as it is today. He narrated that initiating sexual intimacy started gradually from closeness to gifting. The quote below illustrates that:

> It wasn't so easy to tell a girl you want to have sex with her. They would start by giving gifts to the lady, and the lady would know the man wants something. Even from a distance, you will be able to tell. (Osisioma_Female respondent_72 years)

Sexual Practice/Clandestine Sex

In the colonial era, sexual relationships were accepted in the concept of "sexual license." However, pre–civil war sexual practices occurred covertly. It was reported that some adolescents had sex secretly; the girls would go in the company of a younger girl who served as both a guide and a disguise for the senior girl who goes to the partner's house. This was explained in detail in the quotes below:

> Then, some of the girls that were older than me will tell me to follow them somewhere then I was in Primary three. When they are leaving the house, they will tell their parents they are going to their friend's house to collect books or to learn. When we arrive, they will enter the room, while I will remain outside in the next room. I will pretend that I am sleeping. They will cover the curtain when they are done. When they are done, when they try to call me, I will pretend

> that I am sleeping. People had boyfriends and sex back then, but they did it in secret and mostly at night. (Osisioma_Female respondent_72 years)

The sexual practices were mostly consensual sex, and sexual violence rarely occurred. Rape wasn't taken as a serious offence because it hardly occurred, and genuine cases were few. This was vivid in the report by Talbot that:

> Enquiries about rape generally elicited a smile; it was apparently thought that genuine cases were few. . . . As usual, rape was not looked upon as a serious offence. (Talbot 1926, NHB/C/4)

Transactional Sex

In the colonial era, adolescent girls were used to entertain male guests. However, prior to the war, adolescent girls were forced into early marriage and sexual intimacy in exchange for loans, debts, money, land, and favors.

One of the female respondents narrated a family experience to buttress this point, as shown below:

> When my father was very sick to the point of death and there was no money available to treat him, the adopted child of my father was given to a much older man in marriage in exchange for money. It was against her wish, but she went without any objection. After a year, my father died, and my sister came back to the family without any children. (Osisioma_Female respondent_72 years)

She further narrated that any bridal payment made in the event the girl remarried would be refunded back to the former husband. She narrated that:

> Not quite long ago, another man came to marry her and pay back the money owed. She had 12 children for the current husband. In those days, it was common to use girl children in exchange for money, land, or favour. . . . Even if she had not grown for marriage, she would be there till she grew to marry. (Osisioma_Female respondent_72 years)

Sexual Communication

In the colonial era, sexual communication was done through their dressings and hair dressings. However, prior to the civil war, it was reported that some adolescents communicated through writing love letters.

One of the pre-war adolescents reported having married during her early adolescence and having other extramarital affairs during her late adolescence. The quote below summarizes it:

> I got married early at age 15, and later, when I was 19, shortly before the war, I had a boyfriend. . . . We were exchanging love letters. . . . A boy of 4 to 5 years old used to help us exchange the letters. (Osisioma_Female respondent_72 years)

CIVIL WAR TIME (1967–1970)

Early Marriage and Betrothal

Early marriages were reported in the colonial era and pre–civil war times. However, during the war, there was chaos, and this conflict in a way disrupted early marriages and betrothals. This was expressed in these quotes:

> During the war, people were scattered, even people that were betrothed might have migrated to another place. People were more interested how they would be safe. (Aba North_Female respondent_63 years)

In corroboration, another participant averred thus:

> At that time of war, even people that were meant to marry were scattered. Some reunited after the war and got married. It was a tough time. (Obingwa_Male respondent_70 years)

Sexual Initiation

Early sexual initiations were revealed in the colonial period. There was sexual repression in pre–civil war times, and, however, sex became very common during the war.

One of the participants narrated that sex wasn't a regular thing, even shortly before the war commenced:

> Sexual practice at that time wasn't common before the war started. . . . I remember that time when we were in the teachers' quarter. There were about three boys here and four girls living in one room. We didn't know about sex. When we were sleeping, nobody asked us about sexual things, and we didn't know how to sex. (Osisioma_Male respondent_65 years)

However, during the war, having sexual intercourse became more common.

> During the war, having sex became more common. . . . Most of the sex was violent; others were as a result of hunger or protection. (Aba South_Female respondent_61 years)

Sexual Practices During the War—"Civil War Sexual Stories"

Sexual relationships were tolerated in the colonial era under the concept of "sexual license." They occurred secretly pre–civil war times and, however, became commonplace during the war due to the gruesome sexual exploitation perpetrated by the Nigerian and Biafran soldiers.

Sexual Exploitations by Nigerian Soldiers

Nigerian troops captured young girls during the war and afterward, had sexual relations with them against their will. Women who were married were not excluded. One of the participants described this experience in detail:

> Yes, of course, some of the girls were captured by the Nigerian soldiers. . . . The Nigerian soldiers captured some of our sisters and relatives. . . . Even my wife that was pregnant was almost captured. (Aba North_Male respondent_78 years)

Some mothers were threatened; out of fear, they released their daughters to the soldiers. Sexual violence and rape were prevalent at that time. Another participant narrated that:

> When the war ended in 1970, the Nigerian soldiers started capturing young girls and even married women. They will conscript them into their barracks and will sleep with them. They didn't perform any traditional rites on the ladies. Sometimes, when they come to capture the girls and they refuse, they will threaten to kill them. Their mother will beg the girl to follow them to avoid being killed. (Obingwa_Male respondent_74 years)

Another respondent corroborated that:

> The Nigerian army captured the grown-ups. Anywhere they come and see our girls, they will capture them and sleep with them. Because we were small, we were as free as the air.

To avoid being kidnapped by the soldiers, some young females were said to have to disguise themselves as old men and some as insane men. Some married women were said to have abandoned their spouses and followed the army. One of the participants averred that:

> Young girls were disguised as old men because soldiers were sleeping with our girls and women during the war. Without that pregnancy, the soldiers would have captured me. Some married women left their husbands too to stay with the

> soldiers. Some went with the soldiers after the war. (Osisioma_Female respondent_72 years)

Nursing mothers were first not captured, but nursing a baby became a common reason for not being captured, and then the soldiers no longer entertained that as an excuse. According to another participant:

> I heard soldiers were sleeping with our girls and women during the war. After the war, you will hear "apam nwa nka," meaning I have a child in my hand. Because any girl the solders want will sleep with them. For you to resist them, you will say "apam nwa nka." Later, the solders said what be this "apam nwa naka" (come on here give me dure), they subdued them and had sex with them. (Aba North_Male respondent_53 years)

Another participant supported that:

> Well, the soldiers were conscripting women too. Even immediately after the war, the Nigerian soldiers were intoxicated with Igbo girls. Igbo girls were like sacred cows then, and when they saw them, they went wow. They conscripted women, slept with them, married some, left some, and some went along with them. (Aba North_Male respondent_59 years)

Sexual Exploits by the Biafran Soldiers

According to the findings, Biafran soldiers carried away young girls and had sexual intercourse with them. There was no coercion in the bulk of the cases; some young girls and married women went freely to the soldiers, mostly due to hunger and starvation. A male participant narrated that:

> During the war, it is not by force but by money. Yes, girls were dating men who had money, even women themselves. Because of hunger, both married and unmarried women will flock to the soldiers' camp. They give them money and they have sex with them. Their husband knew but could not stop her. If he stops her, hunger will kill them. (Osisioma_Male respondent_65 years)

Furthermore, during the war, Biafra soldiers conscripted young girls and had sexual intimacy with them. Another participant narrated that:

> The Biafran soldiers were conscripting girls during the war while the Nigerians were conscripting girls after the war. . . . Some of the girls gave birth to the soldiers. Some of the girls, when they get pregnant, run away from the soldiers and have their children. The war created an upsurge of illegitimate children. (Aba South_Male respondent_71 years)

According to reports, soldiers who had sexual relations with the young girls died on the battlefield, contributing to their defeat. It was also stated that some soldiers took their concubines to the war front. The respondents viewed sexual freedom as the primary source of defeat at the time. This point was buttered by one of the participants, who said:

> One of the things that brought down Biafra was that, as a result of immoralities, they were capturing girls and keeping them in the camp, whereas by right, women were not supposed to go to the war front. Some soldiers took some of their concubines to the war front. Then, when you sleep with a woman and the next day you go to the war front, you will lose the battle. That was how we started losing the battle. They captured many girls and took them to Dunlop. They were holding a night dance when the Nigerian soldiers came and captured them red-handed and destroyed that place. Sexual immorality contributed to the Biafrans' failure. (Aba North_Male respondent_78 years)

Another participant corroborated that:

> Some carried young girls without force; any Biafran soldier who slept with a lady during the war died on the battlefield; you can never return alive because you have defiled yourself. But Nigerian soldiers carried women to the warfront. (Obingwa_Male respondent_74 years)

Transactional Sex

Adolescent females were exploited to entertain male guests during the colonial era. Prior to the war, adolescent girls were transacted for sex in exchange for favour symbols; however, during the war, sex was transacted in exchange for survival and relief supplies.

One of the participants narrated how his uncle gave his daughter to the Nigerian soldier for sex in exchange for survival. He averred that:

> The Nigerian soldiers captured some of our sisters and relatives . . . Even my wife, who was pregnant, was almost captured. They told them she was a soldier's wife. I was captain then, and I gave her an ID card, but they still refused. My uncle had to give them his own daughter for them to leave my wife alone. If not, they would have killed them. (Aba North_Male respondent_78 years)

The Biafra soldiers, who were placed in charge of giving relief materials to alleviate hunger, used that opportunity to cajole girls into sexual relationships. Sex was transacted in exchange for relief materials. This was narrated as:

> Yes, girls were going to the soldiers so that they had supplies of relief materials as a means of survival, and the officers were also conscripting girls. Some of the

> girls gave birth to the soldiers. Some of the girls, when they get pregnant, run away from the soldiers and have their children. The war created an upsurge of illegitimate children. (Aba South_Male respondent_71 years)

Sexual Communication

Sexual communication was perceived to occur in the form of cultural dressing and hair styling in colonial times. Prior to the civil war, some adolescents were reported to interact via love letters. However, during the war, sexual communications were limited. One of the female respondents gave a detailed account of sexual communication during the war, as illustrated in the quotes below:

> Your parents dare not see you with any boy. At that time, we write love letters and send them to the post office, and you will receive replies too. Even when you have a boyfriend, when you are coming home, you cannot talk about him. No phone, then just letters. Also, when you are going to fetch water, he will see you, and you will talk and chat. That's all. But the war changed a lot of things; it was difficult to communicate. (Aba North_Female respondent_63 years)

POST–CIVIL WAR ERA (1971–1980)

Early Marriage and Betrothal

Early marriages were reported in the colonial era and pre–civil war times. However, during the war, there was chaos. This conflict, in a way, disrupted early marriage and betrothal practices. Post-war, early marriages and betrothals became rare. One of the participants narrated that:

> You will choose whoever you want to marry. Betrothing a girl for marriage at childbirth was uncommon. (Aba South_Male respondent_55 years)

Another person agreed:

> No one chooses my husband for me, I choose him myself. Gone are the days when parents' choice of wives for their sons were done. Anyhow, some still do it, but it is rare. (Obingwa_Female respondent_59 years)

Sexual Initiation

Early sexual initiations were uncovered throughout the colonial era. Prior to the civil war, there was sexual repression; during the civil war, early sexual initiations were common and continued post-civil war. Environmental factors played a role in sexual initiations post-war. One of the participants explained that:

> Sex was mostly for adults, but for teenagers it depends on the environment. When you see your fellow teenager having a boyfriend, you will say, "Let me practice what the other person is doing," but by then it was not too common. (Aba North_Male respondent_53 years)

It was also reported that initiating sex was regarded as tough and that it took time and skills to get a girl to sleep with you. To have a girl sleep with you, you have to be skillful, beg, pet, and wait patiently for it to happen. Another participant reported that:

> It was very tough; you had to be very skillful to get girls to sleep with you. Not now. That is very easy. You can use your phone. (Aba South_Male respondent_55 years)

This was corroborated by another participant who said:

> It was not that common as it is now; when someone asks you to be his friend, you don't have sex just like that. I can remember that the person will ask you, beg you, and pet you before you have sex with him. Then we will be exchanging letters, and then we will find it very difficult to have sex, though we did. Having sex was not that rampant. (Obingwa_Female respondent_59 years)

Sexual Practice

Sexual practices occurred during the colonial period under the concept of "sexual license," occurred covertly prior to the Civil War, and became extremely common and openly practiced during the war. It was alleged after the civil war that there were many brothels, and some adolescents patronized them.

> A survey conducted on youth post-civil war found that there was a surge in brothels' erection, and most of the inmates were mostly adolescents. We counted seven brothels in Aba where half of the inmates were young girls, an average of eighteen years old, although the majority of them were not born in Aba. It was a very tempting situation for young ladies, no matter how enlightened, to fall into prostitution. (Ilogu [1974], R/A/5)

It was reported in the post–civil war period that adolescents who lacked the courage patronized prostitutes; after the war, there was a boom in prostitution, which made having sex easier for men. The details of the sexual practices were explained in the quotes as shown below:

> At that time, you may not have the boldness to meet a girl and ask her for sex. You will meet "ashawo" people. You will go and pay money and sleep with them. (Aba North_Male respondent_53 years)

Transactional Sex

Adolescent girls were used to entertain male guests in colonial times. Used in exchange for material favour, during the pre-civil war, sex was transacted in exchange for survival and relief materials. During and after the civil war, sex was exchanged for money or other material gain. One of the respondents reported that:

> At that time, you may not have the boldness to meet a girl and ask her for sex. You will meet "ashawo" people. You will go and pay money and sleep with them. (Aba North_Male respondent_53 years)

Another respondent stated that:

> If you don't have skills, you have to have money to enjoy sex after the war. (Aba South_Male respondent_55 years)

Sexual Communication

Prior to the civil war, some adolescents communicated through love letters, which were only available during the war. Post–civil war communication was mostly by signs and symbols by the agreed partners and required brain work and accurate timing; this was explained by one of the respondents as shown in the quote below:

> The roof was a means of communication. When I go, I throw a stone three times on the roof of the girl. She will come out and meet you at the place you have agreed to meet. It was really tough then. When you see a girl you like in a place today, tomorrow you will still come to that point to see if you can see that same girl again at the same spot. That time, your brain works. You have to calculate very well. If not, when you go, you will not see her. (Aba South_Male respondent_55 years)

CONTEMPORARY TIMES (1990–TODAY)

Early Marriage and Betrothal

Early marriages were reported in the colonial era and pre–civil war time. They became a rare occurrence in the post–civil war time, and even contemporaneously. A respondent affirms that:

> Early marriages are very rare. A girl must be mature before she can go into marriage. I can't count any of my friends that are married. (Osisioma_Female respondent_18 years)

Sexual Initiation

Early sexual initiations were discovered throughout the colonial era. Prior to the civil war, there was sexual repression. During the civil war, early sexual initiations became very common and continued contemporaneously. Contemporary adolescents narrated that engaging in sexual intercourse early was common, especially among out-of-school adolescents. The participants narrated that:

> Sex is very common; I have friends that talk about it. (Aba South_Female respondent_17 years)

Another participant narrated how they easily discussed sexually related issues:

> Sex is very common when I was in school. We would be discussing sex. Some of us would be watching pornographic movies. (Aba North_Female respondent_17 years)

Another respondent corroborated that:

> Sex is very common these days; some of my friends have had sex. (Osisioma_Female respondent_18 years)

Sexual Practice

Sexual practice occurred under the concept of "sexual license" in the colonial era; covert sex pre–civil war time; sexual coercion in civil war time; proliferation of hotels and patronising commercial sex workers post-civil war; and even in recent times. Contemporary adolescents reported that having sexual intercourse occurred more openly. The common locations were the boyfriend's house, classroom, and brothels. One of the participants averred that:

> Like two of my friends, they didn't even go with their girlfriend. They went out somewhere. . . . Like Ashawo House, that's what they used to call it. I was just coming back from an errand and saw them coming out of there. . . . One was 16 and the other was 19 years old. (Obingwa_Male respondent_17 years)

In corroboration, it was affirmed that:

> My seniors stay in classrooms during prep or when we finish writing our exams and we don't have anything to do, they will arrange to have sex in the classrooms. . . . They do sneak in with phones to communicate. (Aba North_Male respondent_15 years)

Transactional Sex

Adolescent girls were used to entertain male guests in colonial times. Used in exchange for material favours, sex was transacted in exchange for survival and relief materials. In post–civil war times, sex was transacted in exchange for money or other material gain. One of the contemporary adolescents narrated that the transactional sex he experienced was as a result of early emancipation. The adolescents who had been emancipated earlier started a keke business as a means of survival, which in turn became a tool of sexual transaction. He narrated that:

> I have a keke. When I give them a free ride once or twice, they will be looking out for me for a free ride. We call it "free keke." Next time you see them, you will collect their numbers, chat them up, and invite them to the house. When I invited the first girl to the house, I didn't even plan to have sex. She initiated the sex, and we had it. (Obingwa_Male respondent_19 years)

Another respondent reported how he had sex in exchange for a monetary offer. She said that:

> My boyfriend was the first person that dis-virgined me. After that, I started having sex for money. (Osisioma_Female respondent_18 years)

Sexual Communication

Sexual communication was in the form of dressing and hair dressing in colonial times; through love letters in pre–civil war times; sexual communication was limited during civil war times; it took place mostly by signs and symbols post-civil war; and it occurs via mobile phones and social media platforms in recent times. One of the adolescents affirmed that:

> My seniors stay in classrooms during prep or when we finish writing our exams and we don't have anything to do, they will arrange to have sex in the classrooms. . . . They do sneak in with phones to communicate. (Aba North_Male respondent_15 years)

DISCUSSION AND CONCLUSION

The study was conducted to explore the intergenerational patterns of sexual activities among adolescents in Abia state and to explain the possible contribution of an environment event (Nigerian civil war) on the observed patterns in the selected marginalized communities in Abia state. Intergenerational patterns of adolescent sexual activities were traced from the colonial era to contemporary times.

Early marriages and betrothals were common during the colonial and pre–civil war eras. Families betrothed their children as soon as they were born, and this accompanied the exchange of material gifts and favors. After betrothal, the girl underwent female genital mutilation (cutting), and the girl was expected to reside with the boy's family, where her character and personality were observed. At adolescence, the girl would be sent to live with her husband. Other girls who were not betrothed remained in their parents' house until adolescence, when they were of marriageable age. At this point, they would receive a mark before marriage. In a way, this process of receiving marks and marriage helped in maintaining sexual purity among female adolescents, because if a girl got pregnant before then, the marriage was postponed. However, because of the upheaval that accompanied the Nigeria civil war, early marriage and betrothal were somewhat disturbed. This may be due to the fact that most people were more concerned with surviving the conflict, some migrated to other parts of the country to their extended family as a result of the displacement, and some betrothed partners, particularly the males, might have died in the conflict. Due to the challenging economic climate since the end of the civil war and more recently, the majority of men in Abia state choose to achieve financial security before getting married.

Early sexual initiation is allegedly reported to occur as soon as adolescents attain puberty. This is because at attaining puberty, the girl will undergo fattening at the expense of the husband-to-be in her father's compound. During the fattening process, the girl was not allowed to do anything; she was constantly supplied with food and entertained friends, termed the most enjoyable part of the girls' lives. The adolescent boys live in the same house as the other children in the family until they reach puberty, at which point they are forced to move into a separate quarter, or a "bachelor apartment," where they are free to entertain special guests. These different living situations could put adolescents at risk for early sexual initiation. Prior to the civil war, there was sexual repression. The mother placed a high value on the adolescent's premarital chastity and would do everything in her power to ensure that the girl retained it. If the daughter kept her virginity, the mother would get public praise. Virginity came at a hefty price and highly valued. This result was in line with results that girls were supposed to be exceedingly moral and pure, to retain their virginity until marriage, and that a higher importance was put on a girl's virginity in traditional Igbo society. A virgin bride was a source of pride for both her parents and husband (Amadiume, 2005; Uche, 2009; Agbogu & Igbokwe, 2015; Urama, 2019). It was discovered that sex wasn't a common occurrence for male adolescents before the civil war since they weren't thinking about establishing sexual contact. However, because of the gruesome sexual exploitation carried out by the Nigerian and Biafran soldiers throughout the civil war, early sexual initiations were widespread. Early sexual initiation continued after the war and in recent times featuring early sexual debut.

Sexual interactions were acceptable during the colonial era under the concept of "sexual licence" according to findings from archives. In this instance, the mother of a teenage girl consents to the prospective boyfriend's request for sexual intimacy with the girl in exchange for a monetary gift of two shillings. The boy then gives the girl four yams after they have had their sexual encounter. The girl takes care not to get pregnant before she receives the body marks. This sexual licence typically takes place after the potential husband's first visit to the family because she is not supposed to have any sexual intimacy before that visit. This is done with parental consent, especially that of the mother, this practice might in a way restrict sexual freedom among adolescents. Pre-civil war, it was revealed that sex was not a common occurrence as the minds of the adolescents were not focused on sex; most of them were preoccupied with farm work. It wasn't always simple to express your sexual urges to a female; it starts with the expectation that the woman will understand your motives. The concept of sex for love, which is common today, was uncommon then. For example, if a boy meets a girl who catches his eye, he quickly inquires about her parents and if she is already engaged or not. This sexual self-restraint may be attributed to Igbo society's customs, morals, and traditions, which place a premium on dignity and a good name, as the saying goes "*ezi aha ka ego*," "a good name is better than riches."

The narrative of adolescent sexual behavior shifted, particularly in the immediate postwar period, as a result of an environmental catastrophe (the Nigerian civil war) that led to a culture change in the Igbo society. There were stories of sexual exploitations committed by both Nigerian and Biafran soldiers during the conflict. It was revealed that the Nigerian soldiers coerced young females into captivity both during and immediately after the war. Adolescent girls were forcibly conscripted and raped in their barracks throughout the conflict. This conflict-related sexual violence (CRSV) negatively impacted the sexuality norms in the Abia society. After the war, they started capturing young girls and married women; even nursing mothers were not exempt. Some mothers were threatened, so they reluctantly turned over their daughters to the army. Some adolescent girls pretended to be old men, while others pretended to be insane, in order to avoid being captured. According to reports, Biafran soldiers who had sexual relations with women and girls during the war died on the battlefield and perceived to contribute to their defeat and surrender. This was similar to other studies that revealed that there were wartime romances, the rape of girls and women by Nigerian soldiers, many men dying during the war, leaving their wives helpless, children becoming vulnerable to sexual activity, and prostitution being seen as a means of survival, with parents selling off their daughters in exchange for food and protection (Smith, 2005; Akresh et al., 2017). The conflict altered sexuality and made sexual intercourse commonplace in Igbo society, particularly in Abia state, immediately after the war.

Inter-ethnic marriage, which was extremely uncommon in Igbo society, was made more common by the war. Some of the girls who were captured by the Nigerian soldiers came back with their children; some remarried; and a few soldiers who fell in love with the girls subsequently came back and paid the bride price. The soldiers impregnated many young girls during the war, leading to a surge of teenage pregnancy and illegitimate children. According to a study done in Mgbowo, Enugu state, where Nigerian troops committed rapes and fled with some girls who served as saboteurs, sex workers, and "army brides" throughout the fight, the community faced serious threats throughout the war. Some of the "army ladies" returned with children who had been abandoned by their soldier fathers after the war. This was a significant event and marked the beginning of premarital pregnancy, internal elopement among the youth, and the abuse of some sexuality rites and rituals (Nwashindu & Ihediwa, 2016).

Sexual freedom was established during the civil war and persisted after the war. An aftereffect of the conflict was the widespread practice of sexual activity. The war changed the sexual norms. Some participants reported that following the war, having sex was seen as a result of one's abilities, riches, and strategy. Postwar adolescents who engaged in sexual activity were adept at sports like football, which allowed them to easily attract young girls, while others who lacked the courage patronized sex workers. After the war, prostitution became widespread, sparking a sexual explosion. The majority of contemporary adolescents responded that sex was quite common among them and that they openly engaged in sexual conversations with their classmates and watched pornographic movies. The sexual freedom experienced among contemporary adolescents may be as result of modernization, globalization, education, migration, and technological advancements. The Nigerian civil war did not have a direct impact on the recent upsurge of risky sexual exploitations among contemporary adolescents.

Transactional sex cut across all generations of adolescents with different reasons. In colonial and pre–civil war eras, transactional sex occurred in exchange for a loan, debt relief, money, land, or favour. Several adolescent girls were pushed into early marriage in some cases while some girls were kept in the house and used to entertain male visitors. Children born from these liaisons were adopted into the father's family. Some females were given as presents to men in positions of authority by their guardians to gain favour or to secure commercial transactions. These sexual exchanges took place without the girls' consent, putting them at risk of contracting sexually transmitted infections and experiencing unwanted pregnancy because no contraceptive was used during the sexual encounters. During the war, sex was transacted for survival and in exchange for food and protection. As some of the Biafran soldiers were in charge of the relief supplies, sex was more frequently transacted for food, money, and other supplies. This was also similar to a study conducted by Njoku, & Akintayo (2021) where conflicts resulted in transactional sex and sexual violence in northeastern Nigeria. Some young girls and married women gladly went to the soldiers to prevent their children from starving due to widespread famine and poverty. This increased the incidence of sexual exploitations and violence by the soldiers. This corroborates findings that reported Biafran soldiers' wartime relationships and sexual intimacy with some girls (Smith, 2005). These heinous views had never been witnessed in these communities before the war, and they were widely condemned. People's awareness of their sexuality increased after the war and has continued in recent times. Transactional sex became common and is primarily motivated by material acquisition and monetary gain.

Sexual communication varied among different generations of adolescents. The Igbo tradition, which dates back to colonial times and before the war, revealed that girls appeared somewhat naked until puberty, when a piercing of cotton string is worn loosely around the loins. Also, the hairstyles posed a great power of attracting the opposite sex. Although the girls' nakedness symbolized chastity, it could also have been a form of sexual communication, enhancing sexual desire by the opposite sex A similar situation occurred, as reported in a study: Unmarried girls in Afikpo were seen in public wearing only chains of beads around their hips. Being naked or wearing only beads was associated with virginity, chastity, and purity, as clothes were reserved for married women (Ottenberg, 1973). Adolescents during the war communicated by writing love letters and gathering in strategic locations like rivers, farmlands, or bushes where they could talk and unwind. After the war, most communication between parties involved signals and symbols, which required precise timing and mental effort and also writing letters. Adolescents today connect via phone calls, texts, chats, and video conversations because of globalization and technological advancement.

In conclusion, intergenerational patterns of adolescent sexual activities evolved at different times across generations of adolescents. The colonial and pre–civil war eras featured early marriages and betrothals, but this was disrupted during the civil war and had become rare by contemporary times as a result of the harsh economic climate. Early sexual initiations were alleged to occur during adolescence in colonial times, sexual repression was observed prior to the civil war, but during the war, there was a drastic change in the pattern of adolescent sexual activities. The civil-war era featured conflict-related sexual violence, including sexual coercion, sexual freedom, and sexual exploitation perpetrated by the federal troops as well as Biafran officers, whose sole duty was to produce food, particularly after the blockade. This sexual violence and risky sexual exploitations continued post-civil war even in recent times. Transactional sex cut across all generations of adolescents with different purposes: favour and status symbolism (pre-war), sex for survival (during war), and material acquisitions in recent times.

The Nigeria civil war led to the normalization of sexual exploitations among women and young girls, promoted transactional sex as a means of survival, and increased sexual violence and the sexual vulnerability of young girls. This sexual violence and exploitations were mostly perpetrated by the Nigerian soldiers, while the Biafran soldiers maximized the opportunity to satisfy their sexual needs in promise of food, money, relief materials, and protection. The Nigerian civil war had a direct negative impact on adolescent sexual activities in wartime due to the gruesome sexual exploitations, and this continued immediate post-war. The Nigerian civil war had no direct impact on contemporary adolescent sexual activity; factors that may have had a direct impact include globalization, technological advancement, education, and migration. Understanding these trends may aid social interventions to reduce adolescent sexual activities.

REFERENCES

Adetoro, G. (2010). "Socio-economic factors influencing adolescent fertility: Case of Ado-Ota LGA." An unpublished B.Sc. thesis submitted to the Department of Economics, Covenant University, Nigeria.

Agbogu, A. E., & Igbokwe, B. (2015). Gender profiling in Nigeria: the case of the Igbos of southeastern Nigeria. *International Journal of African Society Cultures and Traditions*, *2*(2): 1–10.

Akresh, R., Bhalotra, S., Leone, M., & Osili, U. O. (2012). War and stature: Growing up during The Nigerian civil war. *American Economic Review*, *102*(3): 273–77.

Akresh, R., Bhalotra, S., Leone, M., & Osili, U. O. (2017). *First and second generation impacts of the Biafran war* (No. w23721). National Bureau of Economic Research.

Amadiume, I. (2015). *Male daughters, female husbands: Gender and sex in an African society*. Zed Books, Ltd.

Ayuba, I. I., & Gani, O. (2012). Outcome of teenage pregnancy in the Niger Delta of Nigeria. *Ethiopian journal of health sciences*, *22*(1): 45–50.

Azuike E. C., Iloghalu I. C., Nwabueze S. A., Emelumadu, O. F., Balogun, J. S., Azuike, E. D., Obi, K. M., Enwonwu, K. G., Ebulue, C. C., Obi, D. C., Chikezie, N. I. (2015). Sexual Behaviour Among Senior Secondary School Students in Nnewi North and Nnewi South Local Government Areas of Anambra State. *South-Eastern Nigeria European Journal of Preventive Medicine,* 3(2): 26–33.

Basden, G. T. (1921). *Among the Ibos of Nigeria: An account of the curious & interesting habits, customs, & beliefs of a little known african people by one who has for many years lived amongst them on close & intimate terms*. JB Lippincott Company National Archives Ibadan A1/B.

Bronfenbrenner, U. (1979). *The ecology of human development: Experiments by nature and design*. Cambridge: Harvard University Press.

Curtis, A. C. (2015). "Defining adolescence," *Journal of Adolescent and Family Health:* Vol. 7: Iss. 2, Article 2. Available at: https://scholar.utc.edu/jafh/vol7/iss2/2.

Darroch, J. E., Woog, V., Bankole, A., & Ashford, L. S. (2016). Adding it up: costs and benefits of meeting the contraceptive needs of adolescents.

District office 1922, Southern Province, Tribal Customs and Crimes, with its former Punishments Part 1, Chapter XIII 29/9/65 National Archives Enugu CSE 36/1/10.

District office 1922, Travel, Tribes with their languages and intercourse Part 1 Chapter VII Pg 1227 26/8/65 National Archives Enugu CSE 36/1/6.

Duru, C. B., Ubajaka, C., Nnebue, C. C., Ifeadike, C. O., & Okoro, O. P. (2010). Sexual behaviour and practices among secondary school adolescents in Anambra State, Nigeria. *Afrimedic Journal*, *1*(2): 22–27.

Federal Republic of Nigeria Official Gazette. (2007). "Legal Notice on Publication of the Details of the Breakdown of the National and State Provisional Totals 2006 Census."

Hoiberg, D. H. (2010). Encyclopædia Britannica Ultimate Reference Suite. Chicago: Encyclopædia Britannica.

Ifemesia, C. (1979). Traditional Humane Living Among the Igbo: An Historical Perspective, Enugu. *Nigeria: Fourth Dimension*. National Archives Enugu NHB/C/93.

Ilogu, E. (1974). *Christianity and Ibo culture*. National Archives Enugu.R/A/5.

John, S. P. (2018). 15 examples of culture change; Simplicable. Retrieved from https://simplicable.com/new/culturechange Nigerian Demographic Health Survey (NDHS), 2013.

Njoku, E. T., & Akintayo, J. (2021). Sex for survival: Terrorism, poverty and sexual violence in north-eastern Nigeria. *South African Journal of International Affairs, 28*(2): 285–303.

Nlewem, C., & Amodu, O. K. (2017). Family Characteristics and Structure as Determinants of Sexual Abuse Among Female Secondary School Students in Nigeria: A Brief Report. *Journal of child sexual abuse, 26*(4): 453–64.

Nwankwo, B. O. & Nwoke, E. A. (2009). Risky Sexual Behaviours among Adolescents in Owerri Municipal: Predictors of Unmet Family Health Needs. Journal of African Institute.

Nwashindu, V. & Ihediwa, N. C. (2016). Sexuality and Sex-Related Rituals Among the Mgbowo Women of Awgu Local Government Area, Enugu State. *Nsukka Journal of the Humanities, 24*(2): 1–7.

Olurinola, I. O. (2016). Adolescent Fertility in Nigeria: Trends and, (May).: https://www.researchgate.net/publication/311773394.

Onuche, J. (2014). Marriage and Changing Moral Values in Contemporary Nigeria. *Journal of Sociology and Social Work, 2*(1): 145–55.

Onwuama, M. A.C. & Adepoju, A. (2010). Ethnic and Cultural Determinants of Sexual Behavior among Hausa, Ibo and Yoruba Youths: Implications for Sexuality Education in Nigeria SUB THEME: *Gender, sexuality and culture* www.guttmacher.org/pubs/spib_SSEP.pdf. Classroom Sexuality Education, 231.

Onwubiko, C. A., Ivy, S. C., & Kalu, O. (2015). Determinants of HIV/AIDS Risky Behaviours among Senior Secondary School Students in Aba North Local Government Area, Abia State. *Abia State University Medical Students' Association Journal, 10*(1).

Ottenberg S. (1973). Improvement Associations among the Afikpo Ibo, in Collin M.Turnbull (ed.), *Africa and Change*, New York: Alfred A. Knopf, Inc, 1973, 115.

Reproductive Health/La Revue Africaine de la Santé Reproductive, Vol. 13, No. 1, 135–45. Published by: Women's Health and Action Research Centre (WHARC) Stable.

Smith, D. J. (2000). "These girls today na war-o": Premarital sexuality and modern identity in southeastern Nigeria. *Africa Today*, 99–120.

Smith, D. J. (2005). Legacies of Biafra: Marriage, 'Home People' and Reproduction among the Igbo of Nigeria Africa. *Journal of the International African Institute, 75*(1): 30–45.

Steinberg, L. (2014). *Age of opportunity: Lessons from the new science of adolescence.* Boston: Eamon Dolan/Houghton Mifflin Harcourt.

Talbot, P. A. (1926). *The Peoples of Southern Nigeria: a sketch of their history, ethnology and languages, with an abstract of the 1921 census* (Vol. 3). Oxford University Press, H. Milford. National Archives Enugu NHB/C/4.

Thomas, N. W. (1913). *Anthropological Report on the Ibo-speaking Peoples of Nigeria: Law and Custom of the Ibo of the Asaba district, S. Nigeria.* Harrison and Sons. National Archives Ibadan A1/T74.

Uche, O. O. C. (2009). The socio-religious significance of taboos in Nigeria. *Readings in African thoughts and culture*, 238–57.

UNAIDS. (2014). Estimates. Accessed on August 15, 2018, via https://www.compassion.com/multimedia/unaids-gap-report.pdf.

UNFPA. (2015). Girlhood, not motherhood: Preventing adolescent pregnancy. New York: UNFPA.

United Nation Children's Fund (UNICEF). (2012). Progress for children; a report card on adolescents. eISBN: 978-92-806-463.

United Nations (UN). 2012. Word Population Monitoring: A concise report on adolescent and youth from Department of Economic and Social Affairs Population Division.

Urama, E. N. (2019). The Values and Usefulness of Same-Sex Marriages among the Females in Igbo Culture in the Continuity of Lineage or Posterity. *SAGE Open*, *9*(2): 2158244019850037.

World Health Organization. (2015). Adolescent health. Retrieved from http://www.who.int/topics/adolescent_health/en/.

World Health Organization. (2018). Fact sheet on Adolescent Pregnancy. http://www.who.int/news-room/fact-sheets/detail/adolescent-pregnancy. Accessed August 14, 2021.

Chapter 13

Reversing the Gains?

Exploring the Implications of the Countercurrents of Conflict on Health-Care Access among Fulani in Rural Communities of Southwestern Nigeria

Janet Ogundairo and Ayodele S. Jegede

INTRODUCTION

Conflict between farmers and pastoralists is one of the most pressing and threatening security challenges facing Nigeria in recent times. The conflicts were initially prominent in the northern and central parts of Nigeria but have now extended to the southern part of the country (Higazi and Yousuf, 2018). The crises have socioeconomic implications, as there are records of losses of livelihoods and incomes by both farming and pastoral communities. They have resulted in fatalities, displacements of people, and destruction of property. It was reported in 2019 that more than ten thousand people had been killed in the past decade, with four thousand deaths recorded within the last two years due to farmer–herder clashes in Nigeria (Ilo, Jonathan-Ichaver, & Adamolekun, 2019). Also in 2021, five people lost their lives due to violence while many sustained injuries in farmer–herder clashes in Imeko, the Afon local government area (LGA) of Ogun state (Ogunnaike, 2022). In 2018, the director of department of state services (DSS) in Ondo state reported that the crises have resulted in the destruction of farmlands by pastoralists in farming communities in the state (Sahara Reporters, 2018).

Apart from the loss of lives and properties and the destruction of farmlands, these conflicts also threaten public health. Conflict is a major obstacle to the provision of, and access to, health-care services. People living in areas affected by conflict usually face the challenge of poor health compared to those living in conflict-free areas. Health workers in conflict areas are often targets of attack, harassment, intimidation, and kidnappings and killings while health-care facilities are partially or completely destroyed during conflicts. Ambulatory medical services may be disrupted and/or stopped, especially when health-care officials are not allowed to pass through checkpoints or are even shot at. This further depletes health-care delivery systems that are often weak in developing countries (Rubenstein & Bittle, 2010; Haar & Rubenstein, 2012). These have the consequences of leading to immediate causalities and the denial of opportunities to access health-care facilities and services, especially by those who need them (Haar & Rubenstein, 2012). Vaccination workers in volatile regions in Nigeria were reportedly attacked and killed. This severely disrupted vaccination programmes in those regions (McNeil, 2013).

Conflicts negatively affect health infrastructures in conflict zones. The infrastructures, intentionally or unintentionally, may be damaged, destroyed, or looted by parties engaged in violence/conflict. Health-care facilities as a result of conflict may be shut down or forced to reduce services being provided due to the damage suffered (Fox et al., 2018). This makes it difficult or impossible to treat patients who suffer injuries due to the conflict or those diseases that are indirect consequences of the crises.

Deaths due to non-violence during crises are usually more prevalent than the ones due to violence (Roberts et al., 2004; Coghlan et al., 2006; Degomme and Guha-Sapir, 2010). Degomme and Guha-Sapir (2010) report that non-violent actions during the war in Darfur, Sudan, contributed to the 87 percent of excess deaths of civilian between 2003 and 2008 in Darfur. These non-violent deaths are usually the result of an increase of infectious diseases due to the destruction of health-care facilities, a reduction in the utilization of preventive health services such as vaccinations, the lack of access to potable water, and the scarcity of medication and treatment supplies (Garfield, 2008).

While there have been studies on the causes, trends, dynamics, and consequences of the farmers-herders' crises in southwestern Nigeria, research on the implications of the crises on the provision of, and access to routine health-care services to the pastoralist communities in the region is scanty. Hence, this study explores the implications of the farmers-pastoralists conflicts on health-care access among Fulani in rural communities in southwestern Nigeria. The routine health services in this study include child health (immunization) and tuberculosis diagnosis and treatment. The pastoralists, due to their economic livelihood (cattle herding) and living conditions, are at risk of contracting tuberculosis, which, if left untreated or poorly managed, can result in complications, such as relapse, drug resistance, and even death. The inaccessibility of people to these services could go a long way in reversing the earlier gains made in these routine services and further burden the already-weak health-care delivery system.

CONCEPTUALIZING MARGINALITY/ MARGINALIZATION

Braun and Gatzweiller (2014) see marginality as "the position of people on the edges, preventing their access to resources and opportunities, freedom of choices, and the development of personal capabilities." Marginality occurs when people are disadvantaged or experience barriers in accessing resources needed for them to develop. According to Gatzweiller, Baumuller, Von Braun, and Ladeburger (2011), marginality is "an involuntary position and condition of an individual or group at the margins of social, political, economic, ecological, and biophysical systems, that prevent them from access to resources, assets, services, restraining freedom of choice, preventing the development of capabilities, and eventually causing extreme poverty" The position of marginality, involuntarily occupied by the marginalized person or people, is created by the society.

Marginalization can reflect in disenfranchising people due to their poverty status (Braun and Gatzweiller, 2014), their race or ethnic group (Deuchar, 2009; Slee, 2013), their disability and/or ill health (Slee, 2013), or their religious affiliation (Smith and Barr, 2008). Marginalization can be conceptualized as relating to social exclusion resulting from barriers and unequal opportunities (Messiou, 2012; Petrou et al., 2009); the quest for 'inclusion for all' (Ainscow et al., 2006a; Messiou, 2012; Petrou et al., 2009; Slee and Allan, 2001); specific groups perceived to be especially vulnerable to exclusion and stigmatization (Bottrell, 2007; Petrou et al., 2009); and the need to give marginalized groups a voice (Slee and Allan, 2001).

Social exclusion occurs when there is unequal access to opportunities, benefits, and other resources required to live a decent life. People can be excluded from what are seen as basic needs of man, including water, electricity, health services, and education. Hence to be socially excluded translates to being marginalized. Social exclusion is both a state and a feeling. In a state of being socially excluded, individuals or groups of persons do not have a sense of belonging. There is a feeling of not being valued as members of the community; of being unable to make a tangible contribution to the community; and of not having the rights to access diverse services and opportunities open to other individuals or persons in the society. While others have been marginalized and excluded as a transient experience (Razer et al., 2013), it is part of others' identity and lived experiences (MacLeod, 2013).

This chapter is focused on the marginalization of the pastoralists due to their geographical location, residential/migratory patterns, and their ethnic affiliations, and the impacts on them and on society at large. According to Umar (2006), the pastoralists (who are mostly of Fulani ethnic group) in Nigeria are characterized by marginalization. The environment, both physical and social, in which the Fulani reside and interact exposes them to being marginalized by other people of different ethnic extractions. The physical environments in which the Fulani reside are usually remote from host communities in rural areas. This is usually in order to have access to enough pasture for their cattle and other economic activities (e.g., farming) in which they are involved. The geo-physically disadvantaged locations characterized by poor road networks inhibit their access to resources. They are socially excluded from accessing basic social infrastructures, including schools, electricity, potable water, and good road networks, that could help elevate their standard of living and improve their socioeconomic status.

Fulani/pastoralists have limited access to health services, which are usually designed for settled populations due to their geographical distance (Montavon, Jean-Richard, Bechir et al., 2013). Their settlements can be invisible to health surveillance systems or teams due to their remoteness. Similarly, the mobile pastoralists, due to their mobility, might be unreached by health surveillance teams who are ordinarily not structured to capture mobile populations (Randall, 2015). For the settled pastoralists, they are challenged in accessing health services as the majority of health-care facilities are located in host communities that are far from their settlements. Health workers who are posted to the available scanty primary health facilities in their settlements are usually absent from their duty posts, as there are no motivations or incentives to work in those rural, remote villages.

The social environment, in which the Fulani interacts with the host communities, is unhealthy, thus enhancing their marginalization. According to Ogundairo and Ijimakinwa (2020), the settler's status conferred on the Fulani residing in rural Yoruba communities in southwestern Nigeria formed the basis of them being socially excluded from accessing social amenities such as credit facilities and health and educational facilities in some rural communities in southwestern Nigeria. Recently, they are stigmatized and by extension marginalized in the light of the heightened crises between the herders and farmers in several states in Nigeria. There is heightened animosity towards the Fulani as they are perceived to be criminally minded, wicked, and dangerous. This is not unconnected to the incidences of farm encroachment by cattle, murder, kidnappings, rape, and other criminal activities that have been linked to the Fulani herders. The relationship between them and the Yoruba is rife with animosity, strife, conflicts, distrust, hatred, exclusion, and stigmatization.

The conflicts between the Fulani and Yoruba have public health implications, with mostly the Fulani at the receiving end. The thrust of this chapter is that the Fulani are marginalized and excluded from accessing health services within and outside their settlements as a result of the unhealthy social relationship between them and their hosts.

CONTEXTS

The Fulani in Southwest Nigeria

The southwestern states in Nigeria are made up of Ondo, Ekiti, Osun, Oyo, Ogun, and Lagos states. The dominant ethnic group in these states are the Yoruba-speaking people. The major economies in their rural communities are crop farming, fishing, and trading. Substantial numbers of rural dwellers are farmers. The vegetation is made up of freshwater swamps and mangrove forests (Agboola, 1979), and this has been identified as a major pull factor for the migration of the Fulani from the northern part of the country (Blench, 1994).

The earliest migration of the pastoral Fulani southward, according to Blench, was in the early nineteenth century. He argues that the introduction of the tsetse control measures by the colonial government and the availability of varieties of improved veterinary medicines, demand for cattle, and availability of fertilized, unfarmed land, influenced the movement of the pastoral group into the southwestern part of Nigeria. The Fulani ethnic group has an estimated population of thirty-seven million in Africa, with seventeen million found in Nigeria (Sangare, 2019). They form the majority of the pastoralists in Nigeria (Higazi & Yousuf, 2018). The basis of subsistence of the Fulani includes the sale of milk and dairy products, usually by women, with the men taking on the role of herding (pastoralism) and sales of cattle (Ogundairo & Ijimakinwa, 2019). The cattle, to the Fulani, hold social, cultural, and economic symbols, and thus, they are guarded jealously. Apart from cattle herding, Fulani men in the southwest are also into crop production, while some combine crop production with cattle herding (agro-pastoralism). A few numbers are also into trading (textile, religious materials, etc.).

Previously cooperation and a cordial relationship between the pastoral Fulani and farmers in southwest Nigeria were common and exemplified by farmers leaving post-harvest farm waste for the cattle to forage on, while the cow dung provided manure for the farmers. Conflicts were minor and were settled without escalation. However, this type of symbiotic relationship has disappeared due to the incessant conflicts between the two groups.

Tuberculosis in Nigeria

Tuberculosis (TB) is a global public health problem and a leading cause of mortality in Nigeria (Oluwasanu, Hassan, Adebayo, Ogbuji, Adeniyi, Adewole, Ladipo, Ajuwon, & Ajuwon, 2020). According to the reports of the National Tuberculosis and Leprosy and Control Programme (NTBLCP) in 2019, Nigeria topped the chart of the African countries with the highest burden of tuberculosis. It is also counted among the eight countries accounting for two-thirds of the TB burden globally. In 2020, the WHO reported that Nigeria was the sixth out of thirty highest TB-burdened countries globally and first in Africa in 2018. It was argued that 8 percent of the 4.3 million missed cases globally occurred in Nigeria (Ugwu, Agbo & Ezeonu, 2021).

The TB burden in Nigeria is complicated by multi-drug resistant (MDR) TB, low treatment coverage (NTBLCP, 2017, 2019; WHO, 2018), low case findings; inadequate laboratories; the COVID-19 pandemic, etc. (Adepoju, 2020). A decrease in laboratories confirmed cases of drug-resistant tuberculosis from 2,300 cases that were reported in 2017 to 2,275 cases reported in 2018; while the estimated cases increased from 5,400 to 21,000 in 2018 (Adepoju, 2020). He, however, reported that the country has made significant progress in the percentage of people living with HIV on tuberculosis treatment, which increased from 39 percent in 2017 to 62 percent in 2019.

Similarly, the NTBLCP (2019) submitted that the country has been consistently experiencing an increase in the case identification of TB within four years, spanning from 2017 to 2019. The report further revealed that between 2018 and 2019, the country recorded the highest numbers of case identification since the inception of NTLCP in 1989. There was a 13 percent increase in 2018 from 100,653 to 120,266 in 2019. The report also showed that 77 percent of the United Nations High Level Meeting (UNHLM) target regarding diagnosis and treatment of TB was achieved in 2019, even though there was an extremely low record of people placed on TB-preventive therapy. Another challenge is having a low treatment coverage of 27 percent, as well as a huge number of missing TB cases; that is, failure to follow up in spite of a huge success in case notification.

Improved case findings have been identified as one major way of improving tuberculosis-control efforts (Adepoju, 2020). However, with insecurity challenges rocking the country with incidences of terrorists' attacks, farmers-herders' crises, communal clashes, etc., leading to the displacement of people on either a small or a large scale, case findings will be problematic and thus hinder tuberculosis control efforts in the country.

Pastoralists are at risk of contracting bovine TB (Ibrahim, Cadmus, Umoh, Ajogi, Farouk, Abubakar, Kudi, 2012) due to their interaction with livestock, frequent migration, and consumption of raw milk (Wild, Ali, Bassirou, Tschopp, Barry, & Zinsstag, 2020). However, with the transhumance pattern of the pastoralists coupled with the displacement that some of them are facing as a result of the conflicts between herders and farmers, and by extension the host communities, tuberculosis-control strategies, including case findings and treatments, might be problematic, and thus increase the TB burden and mar the gains in tuberculosis control. It is imperative to treat this as urgent as "one infectious TB case can infect about 15–20 persons per year if untreated" (NTBLCP, 2019).

Childhood Immunization—Prevention Is Better Than Cure

Vaccines are important public health tools (Abdulkarim, Ibrahim, Fawi, Adebayo, & Johnson, 2011) in preventing communicable diseases. Globally, immunization has helped in preventing over two million deaths due to childhood diseases (Odusanya, Alufohai, Meurice, &Ahonkhai, 2008). The Expanded Programme on Immunisation (EPI), a World Health Organisation (WHO) immunisation progamme, was established in 1974 with the aim of making routine immunizations accessible to children for the prevention of childhood diseases (Ophori, Tula, Azih, Okojie, and Ikpo, 2014). It was adopted by the Nigerian government in 1979, and at inception, it was meant to address six killer childhood diseases: tuberculosis, diphtheria, pertussis, tetanus, poliomyelitis, and measles (Ophori, Tula, Azih, Okojie, and Ikpo, 2014). The success of the program led to the inclusion of vaccines for pneumonia, hepatitis B, yellow fever, and meningitis in the immunization package.

According to Ophori et al. (2014), Nigeria achieved the optimum level of coverage of 81.5 percent in the early 1990s. They further stated that the vaccination coverage has been gradual but consistent since the 1990s. The EPI was changed to the National Programme on Immunisation in Nigeria in 1997, and these vaccines continued to be provided freely. Abdulkarim et al. (2011) and Ophori et al. (2014) submitted that the schedule for routine immunization for children in Nigeria is as follows:

> BCG (Bacilli Calmette Guerin): This ought to be administered at birth to children.
>
> OPV (Oral Polio Vaccine): This is scheduled to be administered at birth, and six, ten, and fourteen weeks of age.

DPT (diptheria, pertussis, tetanus): This is to be administered at weeks six, ten, and fourteen.

Measles: This is to be administered at nine months of age.

Yellow fever: This is to be administered at nine months of age.

Hepatitis B: This is to be administered at birth and at weeks six and fourteen.

Vitamin A: This is to be administered at nine and fifteen months of age.

A child is considered to be fully immunized when he or she has been administered BCG, has had three doses of DPT, and has had a minimum of three doses of OPV and one dose of measles vaccine within the first year of birth (Ophori et al., 2014). Immunization helps in preventing dangerous infectious diseases; prevents suffering, disability, and mortality due to diseases; and eases household and health-care systems' expenditures on health (Abdulkarim et al., 2011). The vaccination of children has had a substantial impact on the reduction of mortality due to childhood diseases among children. The WHO (2007) stated there was 60 percent decrease in the global mortality figures due to measles between 1999 and 2005, with the largest gains recorded in Africa, as that continent had nearly a 75 percent yearly decrease in the morbidity and mortality due to measles.

Nigeria has recorded gains in immunization. As earlier stated, the success of the immunization program led to the inclusion of additional vaccines for preventable childhood diseases. In 2010, a total of twenty-one cases of polio from twenty-one local government areas (LGAs) in eight states were recorded in Nigeria. This was a wild departure from the 388 cases that came from 198 LGAs in twenty-seven states in 2009 (Ophori et al., 2014). Nigeria declared itself polio-free on 25 August 2020 (Adebisi, Prisno, & Nuga, 2020).

Despite the gains, Nigeria still faces challenges with vaccine-preventable diseases and low-immunization coverage (Paediatrics Association of Nigeria [PAN], 2021). Challenges to immunization in Nigeria include inadequate funding, religious beliefs and misconceptions, the COVID-19 pandemic, weak access to health services, and conflict (PAN, 2021). Wild, Ali, Bassirou et al. (2020) noted that the positive trends recorded in vaccination coverage in the country might not be reflective of the immunization status of pastoralist communities who are counted among the hard-to-reach populations for health-care services, including vaccination programs. According to Schelling et al. (2007), nomadic populations, as a result of factors such as inadequate health services, challenges in accessing their settlement/camps, and mobility challenges, are frequently missed by immunization campaign teams. Michael, Ashenafi, Ogbuanu et al. (2014) noted that the majority (85 percent) of nomads residing in one of the highest-risk polio areas in Nigeria said they are unable to access the vaccines because their children were absent when vaccination team visited.

METHODOLOGY

The southwestern region in Nigeria consisted of six states (Oyo, Ogun, Osun, Ekiti, Ondo, and Lagos). This study was conducted in selected rural communities in the Ibarapa zone of the Oyo state. The state was selected because it has been a hotspot of farmers-herders' crises in the southwest region. Similarly, the Ibarapa region, out of the four regions in Oyo state, have experienced violent crises between farmers and herders in the state.

The Ibarapa zone is made up of three local governments: the Ibarapa central local government has two towns: Igboora (the LG headquarters) and Idere; the Ibarapa north local government has three towns: Igangan (the LG headquarters), Ayete, and Tapa; while Ibarapa east has two towns: Eruwa (the LG headquarters) and Lanlate. The study was conducted in both the Yoruba and Fulani communities in Ibarapa central and north local government areas. The Yoruba communities that were visited included Igboora, Idere, Tapa, Ayete, and Igangan, while the Fulani settlements included Kajola, Balogun, Akoya, Pakoa, Ekuku, Oniya, and Sekere. Data for the study was collected using primary sources through interviews with pastoralists, farmers, and health workers between 2020 and 2021.Previous fieldwork conducted in the area between 2015 and 2019 by the researcher was also drawn on, along with secondary sources such as academic journals, reports, and newspaper articles.

FINDINGS

Farmers-Herders Conflicts in the Southwest

Farmers-herders' crises in southwestern Nigeria date back several decades, though no accurate date can be cited, but they are usually non-violent. Clashes occur when there is an encroachment of cattle on farmlands, thereby destroying crops and farmlands. Conflicts were usually minimal in occurrence, small-scale and localized, and resolutions were managed through traditional mechanisms that both parties respected. The aggrieved usually lodged complaints with the traditional leaders, and both parties would be invited for dialogue. Once encroachment was established, the pastoralists would be asked to compensate the farmers for the crops or farmland that was destroyed. As a result, these conflicts rarely went beyond the settlements or the communities in which they occurred.

However, the clashes between the two groups have intensified in recent times.[1] It dates back to between 2010 and 2012, but it peaked between 2017 and 2020. The Ibarapa and Oke Ogun areas in Oyo state were particularly affected. This is likely due to the high concentration of pastoralists, who were attracted by vast fertile lands for grazing in these areas. There are also grazing reserves in both areas (Ujorha, 2021). Thus, according to an informant:

> Let's say like 10 years ago was when the matter became unbearable since when the matter has become something the Yoruba could not tolerate again to the extent that it has been happening, but they did not have anyone to help them, but if we look at it from 3 to 5 years ago, it seems the Yoruba do not want the Fulani at all again. This was the period marked with the murder of Dr. Fatai Aborode. Alhaja Subawa was also killed. There were increased incidences of kidnapping, and people were afraid to move around.[2]

Crops destroyed by the cattle that encroached on the farmland are an important source of livelihood. In some instances, herders reportedly go so far as allowing cattle to dry up available water or of polluting with animal dung rivers and streams that a settlement/village or several depend on for survival, thus rendering the water unusable for household use. Farmers, in retaliation for farm encroachment, poison crops on farmlands or water sources, which leads to the death of cattle. Farmers deliberately pour poison on cassava leaves as a form of revenge after experiencing crop damage due to cattle encroachment.

According to a respondent:

> Our farmers, when they realize they are not getting justice when herders encroach on their farms, and to prevent future occurrences, deliberately poison the crops. . . . If there is a herder whose cattle died as a result of consuming the poisoned crops, that means he is guilty of encroaching on the farm.[3]

Cattle die when these leaves are consumed. As a form of retaliation, the herders injure and, in some cases, kill the farmers they meet on farmlands.

Farmers reported that when they confront the herders and accuse them of encroaching on their farms, the herders usually resort to violence, using dangerous weapons such as cutlasses, knives, daggers, and guns to maim and sometimes murder them.

> Some people go to farms because there is nothing they can do except farming. If he is on the farm when the Fulani brings their cows for grazing and he is trying to call the attention of the Fulani man, the man will just say, "What will you now do" since he knows he has power over him. If he talks more than he should, they will just machete him to the extent that they have killed a lot of

people, countless numbers of people have been killed when they confront Fulani for encroaching on their farms.[4]

While mainstream media portrays the Yoruba farmers only as the victims of farm encroachment, harassment, and sometimes harmed and murdered by Fulani herders, it is imperative to note that the Fulani are also victims.

Aside from farm encroachment, the Fulani have also been accused of raping women. This usually occurred when the women are met unaccompanied on farmlands or are on their way to a farm.[5] The herders are also accused of orchestrating kidnappings, which have increased significantly since 2018 (Agbedo, 2021). While the locals point to the Fulani as culprits, findings revealed that the Yoruba and sometimes other ethnic groups have been found to be complicit. Interviews with pastoralists and farmers pointed to some instances where investigations revealed that some cases of kidnappings are orchestrated by Yoruba youth from the communities. These instances however are not reported in mainstream media.

Blockage of grazing routes and encroachment into grazing reserves in a bid to meet the food and shelter needs of a growing population have been identified as one of the factors contributing to the conflicts. Herders have no choice but to graze their cattle, and this, sometimes, leads to farm encroachment when the delineated grazing routes have been blocked and grazing reserves are encroached on. Other factors include desertification and drought; armed conflicts within and outside the country; corrupt law enforcement officers; and the proliferation of small arms and light weapons (SALWs) (Medugu, Majid, & Walter, 2014; International Crisis Group, 2017; Ehiane and Uwizeyimana, 2018; Higazi and Yousuf, 2018). Interviews also revealed that communication barriers between the pastoralists and farmers exacerbate the conflicts.

The incessant conflicts between the farmers and herders have been given ethnic colouration, as they were perceived as subterranean attempts by the Fulani to perpetrate hegemony in Yoruba-speaking states. The increasing violence has strained social cohesion (Ogundairo and Ijimakinwa, 2020) and threatened regional security and stability. Communities in the Ibarapa north local government area evicted the Fulani from their lands. The forceful eviction was avenged by the Fulani, who killed no fewer than eleven people in an Igangan town in June 2021 (Daily Trust, 2021). Presently, there is zero or a very minimal presence of Fulani in communities/settlements/villages in this local government. Any Fulani sighted in this local government is likely to be held with the aim of being murdered. This happened in two instances in May 2022. In one of the occasions, a Fulani was forcefully drawn from a vehicle and killed. Also, a Fulani woman was almost lynched, and she would have been if not for the intervention of one of the locals who pleaded for her release and handed her over to the Fulani in the Ibarapa central local government.

Conflicts have strained the relationship between host and pastoral communities as there exists little or no trust between them. In communities where the Fulani are allowed to stay, interviews with the Fulani revealed that they are not totally comfortable staying and they distrust the olive branch extended by the communities.

IMPACTS OF CONFLICTS ON HEALTH SERVICES

Restricted Movement of Health Workers

Action Against Hunger (ACF) (2021, as cited in Ojeleke et al., 2022) revealed that health workers were attacked, detained, kidnapped, and killed, and health facilities were destroyed, in some communities due to the Boko Haram insurgency (BHI) in northern Nigeria. The awareness that vaccination workers have been reportedly attacked in volatile regions in Nigeria has made immunization teams reluctant to visit some communities in the study area. Though health facilities in Ibarapa communities were not destroyed, because they are located within the host communities where they formed a majority, immunisation teams are often reluctant to go or sometimes afraid of going to Fulani settlements for fear of being attacked.

Health workers who are involved in the diagnosis and treatment of tuberculosis (TB), who are referred to as TB directly observed treatment short course (DOTS) health workers, were also restricted in their operations, due to a fear of being attacked or killed. According to one of the health workers:

> We usually take routine treatments to some pastoralists who do not want to be seen in our clinics for fear of being stigmatized. Even when I notice that a Fulani is coughing incessantly for days sometimes, I approach them, and I give them bottles to collect their sputum sample after I have explained to them what the procedure is all about and the benefits for their health. The majority of our patients in TB clinics are the Fulani with a very good number in treatment. However, due to the conflicts, I had to limit my movement to their settlements for fear of being attacked and killed.[6]

The health worker noted that the fear of being killed or attacked is due to the news that health workers are attacked or killed in states or zones where there are farmer-herder crises or areas affected by the Boko-Haram insurgency. Furthermore, while no health worker has been attacked due to his or her occupational status, there is the belief that they could be attacked in as much as they are Yoruba and not of Fulani stock.

Similarly, mobile drug vendors, who are commonly found in rural settlements and who bridge the gap of inadequate health facilities and health workers in the Fulani settlements, have limited their movements even when they are called by the Fulani to provide health services. While some are frightened of being ambushed, some are reluctant to go because of the fear of being harassed by fellow ethnic members, for being supportive of the enemies of the Yoruba people.

Reluctance of the Fulani to Access Health Care

The Fulani living in settlements outside the host communities who need health-care services are afraid of accessing these services that are mostly located in the host communities for fear of being attacked, injured, or killed by angry locals. One of the pastoralists described the near-impossibility of accessing health-care facilities in town and inviting mobile drug vendors/health vendors to offer services in their settlements.

This occurred at the peak of the crises in Igangan, a period after the self-appointed defender of Yorubaland, Sunday Adeyemo, popularly known as Sunday Igboho, led the community members to evict the Sarkin Fulani and some Fulani from Igangan and neighboring towns and villages in the Ibarapa north local government in January 2021. Herders (who are mostly of Fulani stock) were accused of farm encroachment, kidnapping, murder, rape, and other atrocities by the locals, who believed that the solution to their predicaments is for the eviction of all the Fulani in the location, even though it is not all Fulani who are criminal minded. It is difficult to differentiate between the criminal- and non-criminal-minded Fulani, hence the decision to "throw the bathwater away with the baby." This was their last resolution after they tried to use the police, traditional leaders (from both communities), etc. The locals opined that police and traditional leaders were biased towards the herders when mediating the crises between the herders and the farmers.

Fulani pastoralists who were being treated at the TB DOTS centers in the Ibarapa north local government had difficulty in accessing the host communities for follow-up treatments. This was further exacerbated when the communities evicted the Fulani in large numbers from the local government after the reprisal attacks by the Fulani in June 2021. The Fulani felt they were unjustly treated because they were driven away from lands where they had the right to reside as citizens of Nigerians. There were also reports that attackers during the Sunday Igboho–led eviction in January 2021 carted away money and other stuffs. There were also reports that cows were killed and stolen.

In the Ibarapa central local government, where the Fulani still enjoy some level of acceptance, they showed some reluctance in allowing their children to be immunized. In the words of one of the women:

> If the Yoruba in Igangan (the headquarters of Ibarapa north) could evict the Fulani and kill substantial numbers of Fulani without feeling sober about it, I am reluctant to accept immunization for my children. We, the mothers in this settlement, have resolved to shun vaccination for our children even if the vaccination team comes here. Who knows the extent to which they can go? We know some Yoruba do not want us to stay. Our staying here is not pleasant to them. Such people can poison our children under the guise of immunization. We have had meetings not to accept any health interventions from the host communities for now.[7]

The distrust between the two ethnic groups due to the conflict and its aftermath has resulted in women from the pastoral settlement in this local government shunning public health-care services even when they are made available.

Disruptions of Routine Health Services

Infectious disease control, eradication strategies, and vaccination campaigns often experience disruption in conflict-ridden settings (Footer and Rubenstein, 2013). In the study area, the reluctance of TB patients to access health-care facilities in host communities, as well as the hesitancy on the part of health officials to offer diagnosis and follow-up services in Fulani settlements due to the fear of being attacked, have led to the disruption of TB diagnosis and treatment. Health workers who were interviewed submitted that the majority of those who are on treatment missed their appointments as a result of the conflicts.

There is a challenge in reaching our patients (Fulani) who are being treated for tuberculosis. It has been challenging following up with old patients and getting new ones as the conflicts between the farmers and herders become more pronounced. This got worse following the forceful eviction and mass exodus of the Fulani from our communities. A very good number of our patients are Fulani, and we have lost them to follow-up as a result of the crises.

The migration and resettlement experiences of displaced persons, as well as accessing health-care services (including routine health services, e.g., TB services), are usually daunting and challenging. According to Bornemisza et al. (2010) and the World Health Organization (WHO) (2017), victims of conflict in transit, internally displaced persons, find it difficult to access needed medical services, thus leading to disruptions in vaccination and tuberculosis treatments. Similarly, the displaced population, while in search for where to settle, might be overlooked for health-surveillance systems that are primarily designed for stationary populations.

The TB DOTS officer who was interviewed noted that:

> There is no doubt that several of our Fulani patients who have migrated en-masse from our communities will experience disruption in accessing their TB services. While migrating, they will not think of their TB treatment because their survival and that of their household will be of paramount importance when compared to TB. Our TB patients before the eviction and mass migration were above 100. We do not have many patients again because the majority are Fulani. It is unfortunate that the dispersal of these people has reverted the earlier gains we have made regarding diagnosis and treatment of TB.

The inability of this displaced population to access routine services, including screening for TB and immunizations, could hinder the effective control of TB and vaccine-preventable diseases among children. In Nepal, the disruption in the uptake of tuberculosis diagnosis and treatment led to the prevalence of tuberculosis (Tiwari et al., 2005). Disruption of TB treatment has been identified as one major factor contributing to relapse, treatment failure, ongoing transmission, drug resistance, and even death among people living with tuberculosis. This will greatly mar the disease control of the government and affect the country's goal of reducing the health burden due to these diseases. Hence, programs aimed at controlling these diseases should endeavor to innovate strategies to reach this population with various disease-control interventions.

CONCLUSION

Conflicts create barriers for health workers who are unable to provide necessary health-care services, and for the sick members of society because they are then unable to access health-care services, including necessary health-care infrastructures. The study concludes that the conflicts between farmers and herders have adverse effects on the access of the Fulani people to immunizations/vaccinations and tuberculosis treatments in rural communities in southwestern Nigeria. There is less chance that children from pastoral communities in conflict areas will be able to access immunizations. This has implications on the public health and increases the health-care burden due to vaccine-preventable diseases spreading in children under the age of five in Nigeria. In the face of perceived danger, and due to conflict-induced migration, there is less chance that children from pastoral communities in rural communities will be able to access immunization. Similarly, there will be a disruption in tuberculosis diagnosis and treatment for pastoralists affected by tuberculosis. All these things could mar and reverse the earlier recorded gains in vaccination and immunization, as well as the prevalence of tuberculosis, and thus it could increase the country's public health burden.

The government and other stakeholders need to properly manage conflicts to avert poor health outcomes, especially as the existence of conflicts and crises can have adverse effects on public health. Public health is threatened during times of conflict, and as such, strategies and policies at addressing the trends and dynamics in conflicts need to include adaptation to, and provision of, public-health palliative and remedial measures, a situation that will bridge gaps that may occur in health-care provision and access in times of crisis.

ACKNOWLEDGMENT

The main data for this manuscript was collected during the PhD fieldwork conducted by the first author. The French Institute for Research in Africa (IFRA)—Nigeria is appreciated for providing a small fieldwork grant for the thesis.

REFERENCES

Abdulkarim, A.A., Ibrahim, R.M., Fawi, A.O., Adebayo, O.A., & Johnson, A'WBR. (2011). Vaccines and immunization: The past, present and future in Nigeria. *Nigerian Journal of Paediatrics*, 38(4):186–94.

Adebisi, Y.A., Prisno, D.E., & Nuga, B.B. (2020). Last fight of wild Polio in Africa: Nigeria's battle. *Public Health in practice*.

Adepoju, P. (2020). Nigeria's widening Tuberculosis Gap. *Lancet Infectious Diseases*, 20:29.

Aderinoye-Abdulwahab, S.A. & Adefalu, L.L. (2012). Pastoral communities in Nigeria: Another case of marginalization. Paper presented at the 56th AARES Annual Conference, Fremantle, Western Australia.

Agbedo, O. (2021, January 30). Charting the way forward for age-long conflict. *Guardian*. 30 January. https://guardian.ng/saturday-magazine/herders-farmers-clash-charting-way-forward-for-age-long-conflict/.

Agboola, S.A. (1979). *An agricultural atlas of Nigeria*. Oxford University Press.

Blench, R. (1994). The Expansion and Adaptation of Fulbe Pastoralism to Subhumid and Humid Conditions in Nigeria. *Cahiers d'Études Africaines*, 34: 197–212.

Bornemisza, O., Ranson, M.K., Poletti, T.M., & Sondorp, E. (2010). Promoting Health Equity in Conflict-Affected Fragile States. *Soc Sci Med*, 70(1): 80–88.

Coghlan, B., Brennan, R., Ngoy, P., Dofara, D., Otto, B., Clements, M., and Stewart, T. (2006). Mortality in the Democratic Republic of Congo: A Nationwide Survey. *Lancet*, 367 (9504): 44–51.

Degomme, O., and Guha-Sapir, D. (2010). Patterns of mortality rates in Darfur conflict. *Lancet*, 375 (9711): 294–300.

Deuchar, R. (2009). *Gangs, marginalised youth and social capital*. Dunedin Press.

Footer, K.H.A., & Rubenstein, L.S. (2013). A human rights approach to health care in conflicts. *International Review of Red Cross,* 95(889): 167–87.

Fox, H., Stoddard, A., Harmer, A., & Davidoff, J. (2018). Emergency trauma response to the Mosul offensive, 2016–2017: Review of Issues and Challenges. *Humanitarian Outcomes*, 10.

Garfield, R. (2008). The epidemiology of war. In B. Levy and V.W. Sidel (eds). *War and Public Health.* American Public Health Association.

Gatzweiler, F., Baumüller, H., von Braun, J., Ladeburger, C. (2011). Marginality: addressing the root causes of extreme poverty. ZEF working paper 77, Center for Development Research, University of Bonn, Bonn.

Haar, R.J., & Rubenstein, L.S. (2012). *Health in post-conflict and fragile states.* United States Institutes of Peace.

Higazi, A. & Yousuf, A. (2018). *From cooperation to contention: political unsettlement and farmer-pastoralist conflicts in Nigeria.* Conciliation Resources.

Ibrahim, S., Cadmus, S.I.B., Umoh, J.U., Ajogi, I., Farouk, U.M., Abubakar, U.B., & Kudi, A.C. (2012). Tuberculosis in humans and cattle in Jigawa State, Nigeria: Risk factors analysis. *Vet Medicine International.*

Ilo, U.J., Jonathan-Ichaver, L., & Adamolekun, Y. (2019, January 13). The deadliest conflict you've never heard of: Nigeria's cattle herders and farmers wage a resource war. *Foreign Affairs.* https://www.foreignaffairs.com/articles/nigeria/2019-01-23/deadliest-conflict-youve-never-heard (accessed November 20, 2020).

McNeil Jr., D.G. (2013, February 8). Gunmen kill Nigerian polio vaccine workers in echo of Pakistan attacks. *New York Times.* http://www.nytimes.com/2013/02/09/world/africa/in- nigeria-polio-vaccine-workers-are-killed-by-gunmen.html?_r=0.

Michael, C.A., Ashenafi, S., Ogbuanu, I.U. et al. (2014). An evaluation of community perspectives and contributing factors to missed children during an oral polio vaccination campaign—Katsina State, Nigeria. *J Infect Dis.*, 210(suppl 1): S131–S135.

Montavon, A., Jean-Richard, V., Bechir, M. et al. (2013). Health of mobile pastoralists in the Sahel—assessment of 15 years of research and development. *Trop Med Int Health*, 18: 1044–52.

National Tuberculosis and Leprosy Control Programme (NTBLCP). Annual Review Meeting (2017).

National Tuberculosis and Leprosy Control Programme (NTBLCP). (2019). 2019 Annual TB Report. Federal Ministry of Health, Nigeria.

Odusanya, O.O., Alufohai, E.F., Meurice, F.P., & Ahonkhai, V.I. (2008). Determinants of Vaccination Coverage in Rural Nigeria. *BMC. Public Health*, 8: 381.

Ogundairo, J.A., & Ijimakinwa, F. (2020). Pastoralism and Politics of Exclusion in Ibarapa, Oyo State, Nigeria. *African studies*, 79(4): 428–43.

Ogunnaike, J. (2022 January 15). Five killed, many injured in fresh farmer-herder clash in Ondo. *Vanguard.* https://www.vanguardngr.com/2022/01/five-killed-many-injured-in-fresh-farmers-herders-clash-in-ogun/.

Ojeleke, O., Groot, W., Bonuedi, I., & Pavlova, M. (2022). The Impacts of Armed Conflicts on Health Care Utilization in Northern Nigeria: A Difference—in—Differences Analysis. *World Medical and Health Policy*, 1–41.

Oke, J., Dalibi, A., Ojuola, B., & Owuamanam, J.A. (2021, June 7). 15 killed at Igangan, four months after sack of Fulani settlement. *Daily Trust.* https://dailytrust.com/15-killed-at-igangan-four-months-after-sack-of-fulani-settlement.

Oluwasanu, M.M., Hassan, A., Adebayo, A.M., Ogbuji, Q.C., Adeniyi, B.O., Adewole, D.A., Ladipo, O.A., Ajuwon, G.A., & Ajuwon, A. (2020). General and tuberculosis-specific service readiness in two states in Nigeria. *BMC Health Services Research*, 20:792. https://doi.org/10.1186/s12913-020-05626-3.

Ophori, E.A., Tula, M.Y., Azih, A.V., Okojie, R. and Ikpo, P.E. (2014). Current Trends of Immunization in Nigeria: Prospect and Challenges. *Tropical Medicine and Health,* Vol. 42, No. 2, 2014, 67–75. doi: 10.2149/tmh.2013-13.

Randall, S. (2015). Where have all the nomads gone? Fifty years of statistical and demographic invisibilities of African mobile pastoralists. *Pastoralism* 2015: 5: 22.

Roberts, L., Lafta, R., Garfield, R., Khudhairi, J., & Burnham, G. (2004). Mortality Before and After the 2003 Invasion of Iraq: Cluster Sample Survey. *Lancet,* 364(9448): 1857–64.

Rubenstein, L.S., and Bittle, M.D. (2010). Responsibility for Protection of Medical Workers and Facilities in Armed Conflict. *Lancet,* 375(711): 329–40.

Sangare, B. (2019). Fulani people and Jihadism in Sahel and West African countries. Foundation Pour La Recherche Strategique, March 2019. https://www.frstrategie.org/en/programs/observa-toire-du-monde-arabo-musulman-et-du-sahel/fulani-people-jihadism-sahel-and-west-african-countries-2019.

Schelling, E. et al. (2007). Human and animal vaccination delivery to remote nomadic families, Chad. *Emerg Infect Dis*, 13: 373–79.

Slee, R. (2013). The labelling and categorisation of children with emotional and behavioural difficulties: A cautionary consideration. In: Cole, T., Daniels, H. and Visser, J. (eds.). *The Routledge International Companion to Emotional and Behavioural Difficulties [Routledge Handbook].* Routledge, 15–21.

Smith, R. and Barr, S. (2008). Towards education inclusion in a contested society: From critical analysis to creative action. *International Journal of Inclusive Education,* 12(4): 401–22.

Tiwari, S.K., Sitthi-Amorn, C., Wang, J.L, Kasetjaroen, Y., & Love, E.J. (2005). Prevalence of TB and Service Utilization in Conflict Affected Areas of Nepal. *Journal of Nepal Health Research Council*, 3(1): 45–57.

Ujorha, T. (2021, April 3). Sarkin Fulani: Strange turn of events after 50 years. *Daily Trust*, 35.

Umar, A. (2006). The teacher education curriculum and the world of work: A study of teachers of disadvantaged children in Nigeria. *Teacher and Teacher Education,* Vol. 22(7), October 2006, 777–87.

Von Braun, J. & Gatzweiller, F.W. (2014). An overview and implications for policy. In Von Braun, J. & Gatzweiller, F.W. (eds). Marginality: Addressing the nexus of poverty, exclusion and ecology. Springer, 1–23.

Wild, H., Ali, S.M., Bassirou, B., Tschopp, R., Barry, M., and Zinsstag, J. (2020). Mobile pastoralists in Africa: a blind spot in global health surveillance. *Tropical Medicine and International Health*, vol. 25, no. 11: 1328–31. doi:10.1111/tmi.13479.

World Health Organization (WHO). (2007). Measles. WHO Fact sheet N°286. WHO.
World Health Organization (WHO). (2018). Guidelines on management of drug resistance TB. WHO.
World Health Organization. (2019, September 5). *One Year after Nigeria Emergency Declaration.* www.who.int/news-room/feature-stories/detail/one-year-after-nigeria-emergency-declaration-.
World Health Organization (WHO). (2020). Tuberculosis Fact Sheet. WHO, Zurich.

NOTES

1. In northern Nigeria, the use of arms and ammunitions by both farmers and pastoralists have been reported. The main group noted for the heavy use of weapons in the southwest are the pastoralists. However, small arms use is becoming more common among the farmers in the southwest as a form of defense and as a weapon for undertaking reprisal attacks.

2. Interview conducted in September 2021 with a female farmer in Igangan, Ibarapa north LGA, Oyo state.

3. Interview conducted in September 2021 with a farmer in Igangane, Ibarapa north LGA, Oyo state.

4. Interview conducted in September 2021 with a female farmer in Igangan, Ibarapa north LGA, Oyo state.

5. Ibid.

6. Ibid.

7. Interview conducted with health worker in August 2021.

Chapter 14

Livelihood and Health Challenges in Farm Settlements in Akwa Ibom State, Nigeria

Nsikanabasi Udofia Wilson, Moses Idongesit Peters, and Aniekan Etim Bassey

INTRODUCTION

Health-care service is a major challenge within farmers' settlement areas in Akwa Ibom State. Though they are food-producing communities, good health remains a great supplementary factor to food and enhances effective food production. Titus, Adebisola, and Adeniji (2015) posit that sound health is a fundamental requirement for living a socially and economically productive life, and poor health inflicts great hardships on households, including debilitation, substantial monetary expenditures, loss of labor, and sometimes death. The nature of work and labor available in the farmers' settlement areas is such that it requires good health-care attention from time to time. Asenso-Okyere, Chiang, Thangata, and Andam (2011) observed that the health status of adults affects their ability to work and thus underpins the welfare of the household, including the children's development. Bad or poor health affects productivity, especially at old age, and it sometimes leads to untimely death when there is no access to health-care services. Good health-care provision and accessibility enhanced good health and makes life worth living (Asenso–Okyere, Chiang, Thangata, and Andam, 2011).

The World Health Organization (WHO, 1948) conceptualizes health as a state of complete physical, mental, and social well-being and not merely the absence of disease or infirmity (Innocent, Uche, and Uche, 2014). According to Kajang (2004), health-care delivery in Nigeria operates in the three tiers of government: local, state, and federal. This accounts for the disparities in quality, availability, cost, and level of utilizations in the health sector in Nigeria. Nigeria has over 70 percent of her inhabitants living in rural communities, yet the area has not attracted sufficient health facilities/projects that would substantially improve the health needs of the rural dwellers (Ama, Okeme, and Chia, 2015). This has posed a serious concern for the rural farmers. According to Hamid, Sadique, Ahmed, and Molla (2005), many low-income countries, Nigeria included, have not been able to meet the basic health-care needs of their people, especially those in the rural areas. Olayiwola (1990), cited in Ama, Okeme, and Chia (2015), posited that the health-care system in Nigeria and the health status of Nigerians are in a horrendous state. Health-care delivery in rural areas of Nigeria is still in a state of great concern, especially in the area of professionals and the availability of drugs for rural usage. Quack health-care service providers have made good exploits of the rural dwellers, and therefore they contribute to the bad health condition of most of the rural dwellers.

Bunor (2004) posits that the dimensions of distance to services, such as travel time, waiting time, appointment time with doctors, and nature of the means of transport, have an effect on the utilization of health facilities. Anum (2015) argued that poverty and illiteracy can also affect the use of health services. People may lack enabling resources, and because of the high rate of illiteracy, they might not perceive the need for health-service use, especially rural people, resulting in the use of unscientifically tested traditional medicine, some of which has negative health implications (Anum, 2015). According to Okon (2001), overcrowded wards; long wait times for patients; poorly trained, overworked and underpaid health-care personnel; a dearth of specialist doctors due to brain drain; a lack of increased spots for specialist training; and the loss of revenue to countries such as India, the UK, and the United States, which attract Nigerians to "better health care" and coin the term *health tourism* to their benefit. These have led to the detriment of public health-care services and their utilization in Nigeria. The above listed facts revealed the need for a revamp of the health-care system in Nigeria (Okon, 2001).

Since the majority of rural farmers do not have access to mechanized systems of farming or agricultural practices, their farming activities become strenuous and require much energy, and they need good health for effectiveness and efficiency. The nature of the work within the farm settlement areas poises a demand for well-funded and well-equipped health-care facilities if any pragmatic approach toward provision of health-care services for rural farmers are to be embarked upon by any institution or organization. When there is no health-care facility in such areas or close to the farmers, alternative medicine becomes the hope of the rural farmers, else the poor health status of the farmers affects their productivity in food production, especially when they utilize non-mechanized agricultural practices. The level of accessibility of health-care services by farmers in farmers' settlement areas in Akwa Ibom State depends on the state of the health-care services in Nigeria. Access to health-care services is a multidimensional process involving the quality of care, geographical accessibility, availability of the right type of care for those in need, financial accessibility, and acceptability of the service (Peters, Garg, Bloom, Walker, Brieger, and Rahman, 2008). The utilization of health-care services is related to the availability, quality, and cost of services, as well as socioeconomic structure and personal characteristics of the users (Onah, Ikeako, and Iloabachie, 2009). Accessing health care in rural areas is confounded by problems such as insufficient health infrastructure, the presence of chronic diseases and disabilities, and socioeconomic and physical barriers (Ricketts, 2009).

Most of the health-care facilities in Nigeria have been concentrated in the urban centers, such that the rural areas are left out of health-care services distributions. The absences or low number of health-care facilities in the majority of the rural areas in Nigeria have contributed to the poor health status of the rural dwellers, and it affects their level of usage of health-care services. Ajilowo and Olujimi, (2007) noted that most of the health infrastructural facilities are concentrated in urban areas, to the neglect of rural areas, and the few health facilities located in the rural areas are not in good states and do not function effectively. According to Okon (2001), the health system in Nigeria is still facing serious challenges, like inappropriate budgetary allocations, poor infrastructure in the public health facilities, a lack of drugs, an uneven distribution of health facilities, and a lack of qualified medical personnel. Farmers' settlement areas in Akwa Ibom State are located within the rural areas of the state. The absence of health-care facilities is a key characteristic of these rural areas. Women and children are vulnerable to health problems. Most men suffered health problems due to old age, and traditional medicines replace orthodox medical practices in these communities. Against this backdrop, this chapter seeks to examine the level of availability of health-care services; available options, coping strategies, and intervention programmes in these farm settlement areas.

METHODOLOGY

Study Location and Research Design

The study was carried out in the Isohidim and Akpansung farm settlement areas, in the Ibeno and Esit Eket local government areas, Akwa Ibom State, in the southern region of Nigeria. The areas have no health-care centre. The inhabitants of these communities are multiethnic groupings found within Akwa Ibom State. These multiethnic human groupings include Ekid, Annang, Ibibio, and Oro. The research design was non-experimental and was concentrated on a qualitative investigation of the level of availability of health-care services, available options, coping strategies, and intervention programs among farm settlement areas' dwellers in the Ibeno and Esit Eket local government areas of Akwa Ibom State.

Sampling

The study population included youth (both males and females), men, and women of eighteen years and above. Study participants were randomly selected and engaged in the study. Females were the majority of the gender class, while males were the fewest in gender structure of the study participants. Within the period of study, participants were randomly selected based on availability.

Study Instrument

Interview schedules were used for the study with open-ended questions based on the subjects of health care among the rural dwellers within the farm settlement areas. Participant observation was also adopted by the researchers for the study, with focus group discussion (FGD). Interviews were conducted in the Ibibio language, which serves as the general language used among the people.

Data Management

Data collected were transcribed in English language for easy analysis and proper presentation of findings of the study for general consumption. Data were analyzed thematically in line with the themes of the study objectives. Thematic analysis was adopted for a qualitative analysis of the findings with extracts of some of the key responses of some of the study participants.

RESULTS

Anderson's model of health care utilization was adopted for the study. According to Okumagba (2011), Anderson (1983) grouped in a three-sequence cluster of factors, which are predisposing, enabling, and need factors that are capable of influencing health behaviors. This model explains the factors that influence the needs for health-care services by the people, the factors that permit their demands, and the accessibility of health-care services, the essential factors that prompt their utilizations. The model is illustrated in figure 14.1 below.

The analysis of data gathered through recorded interviews and participants' observations sought to identify key themes and variables (Bryant and Charmaz, 2007, in Philips, Ononokpono, and Udofia, 2016). Qualitative analysis was used for the narratives to explain the level of availability of health-care services; available options; coping strategies; and health-care intervention programmes in the farm settlement areas.

Availability of Health-Care Services

Ricketts (2009) posits that accessing health care in rural areas is confounded by problems, such as insufficient health infrastructure, the presence of chronic diseases and disabilities, and socioeconomic and physical barriers. According to Aghion, Peter, and Fabrice (2010), health-care access and utilization are of major interest to rural development; this is because they are vital elements of well-being and components of human capital. According to Onokerhoraye (1999), overt attention has not been paid to equity in the planning and distribution of health-care facilities over the years in the country. Public and private health-care facilities are sporadically provided in many rural areas within the country (Onokerhoraye, 1999). These scholarly positions explain the status of the Isohidim and Akpansung farm settlement communities. Through participant observation, it was observed that none of these communities has a single-room health-care center. There was no chemist or medical practitioner in these farm settlement areas. This contributes to the difficult health-care situation experienced by the farmers and other dwellers within these communities. The majority of the study participants lamented their helpless health-care conditions. Many narratives were recorded on the many difficult health-care experiences of the people.

One of the female participants from Akpansung community in her narratives explained that:

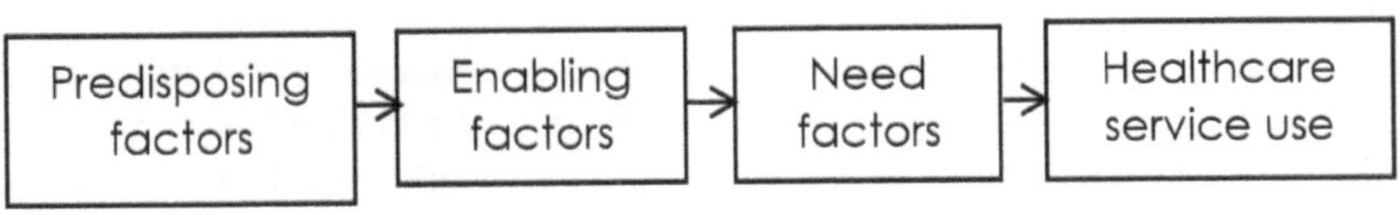

Figure 14.1. Anderson's health-care utilization model. Adapted by the authors from Anderson, R. (1983). Health Services Utilization: Framework and Review. *Health Services Research*, 3: 184–99.

> We are really suffering here. We don't have any health care center here, and we don't have one that is close to us. We struggle to help our children to live anytime they are sick. We struggle to see how they can survive from sickness through the use of herbs and roots we can find here. If it is not for one man (Mr. Abiata) who is a specialist in roots and herbs, we would have lost almost all our children by now.

The physical environment of some rural areas contributes to the neglect of the allocation of health-care facilities. According to Titus, Adebisola, and Adenyi (2015), such regions with difficult terrain and physical environments are often neglected. The Isohidim and Akpansung communities are physically located along the riverine area in Akwa Ibom State. Their locations have positioned them far from the nearby towns of Ibeno and Eket. This situation constitutes a barrier to health-care service accessibility by the people. The majority of the study participants, in their narrative during focus-group discussion, expressed their ordeal in accessing health-care services outside their settlement areas.

Another female participant, during a focus group discussion at Akpansung community, stated that:

> The hospitals are far from us. We have one at Ukpeikang and Emmanuel hospital at Eket. We hardly go there because the distance between our community and these hospitals is very much. Sometimes our women will have to give birth by the water side, especially those who cannot cross the wooden bridge under labor. So, they will weep and lie by the waterside to deliver their babies, and all the women in this community will join efforts together to see how to save the baby and the mother before they can be taken to the hospital either at Ukpenikang or at Eket. We are really suffering because of the lack of health-care facilities here. Some time we lost our children because, before you think of getting them to the hospital, they died on the way, and the parent will bring the corpse back for the entire community to mourn.

A female participant from Isohidim during her interview narrated that:

> We have lost our people to death because the hospitals are far from us. In most of those cases, they died on the way to the hospitals. If we have at least a one-room health-care center here, we will not lose our brethren to death as we have in recent times.

Good health can contribute to an increase of food production by farmers who live in the rural areas and do not have access to mechanized farming techniques. Since much energy is needed for hard farmwork, good health becomes a prerequisite for the ability to do farmwork and have good agricultural production. In their narratives, the majority of the study participants believe that good health contributes to a good working farm day and a bountiful harvest, and a poor health status contributes to poor agricultural production.

One of the male participants from Isohidim in his narrative explained that:

> We need to be sound in our body to be able to do farmwork. You cannot work in the farm if you are not feeling well in your body. Farmwork is not an easy job; it requires a lot of energy, and it takes sound health to do that. We would have produced more foodstuffs if we can have health-care services to attend to our health needs when we are sick. But people can just lie for days and sometimes weeks to see how to recover from sickness through the use of herbs and roots. This affects our productivity.

The Isohidim and Akpansung farm settlement areas are neglected in health-care facility distributions. Their locations may contribute, but the health of every citizen should be the concern of every government. The well-being and health condition of the people living in these areas are left in the hands of the people as rural communities. The distance between the next available health-care facility and these communities is far enough to discourage patronage of the health-care facilities.

Available Health-Care Options and Coping Strategies

According to Anum (2015), the geographical distribution of health-care facilities may also influence the utilization of health clinics. In a comparison of the distribution of hospitals between urban and rural areas in Nigeria, Anum opined that whereas approximately 80 percent of the population of the selected states lived in rural regions, only 42 percent of hospitals were located in those areas. The maldistribution of physicians was even more marked, because few trained doctors who had a choice wanted to live in rural area. Many of the doctors who did work in rural areas were there as part of their required service in the National Youth Service Corps, established in 1973 (Anum, 2015). This position of Anum (2015) is an indication of the nature of available health options in the rural areas. In the Isohidim and Akpansung rural farmers' settlements, no medical or health-care service provider was found at the time of this fieldwork in 2018. The question of available options of health-care services was not to include any primary, secondary, or tertiary orthodox medical services to be provided by the local, state, or federal governments. The majority of the study participants in their narratives explained the absence of health-care services from any orthodox health-care service providers as an available option for health care in these communities.

One of the male participants from the Isohidim farmers' settlement in his narratives explained that:

> There is no conventional trained health-care provider in our community. We do not have even a private medical businessperson in this community. We do go to Mkpanak to buy drugs and keep them at home. If you don't buy medicines and keep them and your child gets sick in the night, you may lose him/her. Some people have been losing their loved ones to death because no health-care service is available here as an option.

A female participant from Akpansung in her narratives explained that:

> We do not have white man medicines here. Some people do go to Mkpanak, Ukpenikang, or Eket to buy medicines. We are suffering because we do not have access to a health-care facility here.

Due to the non-availability of health-care services, the people have resolved to depend on few affordable drugs from neighbouring communities and traditional medicines served from roots and herbs by one of the residents of the communities. The majority of the participants, in their narratives, explained that they often depend on herbs and roots as traditional medicines for a health-care option.

One of the male participants, during the focus group discussion at Isohidim, narrated that:

> Herbs and roots are our hope apart from God here. We depend on herbs, and they have not failed us because God knows that nobody cares about the situation of farmers in Isohidim, but we supply this part of the state with food, wine, firewood, timber, and charcoals.

When what is needed and expected is not available, the people turn to what hope can provide. The people of the Isohidim and Akpansung farmers' settlements have turned to hope in God for help in times of health crises. The majority of the study participants agreed that God is their available option for help in times of health crises. Though they trust in divine healing, they ceased not to seek health-care services when they could afford to go all the way to get it.

A female participant from Akpansung community during a focus group discussion stated that:

> The all-available option for us in terms of health care is God. We trust God to give us divine healing when we are in need. He is the one that protects us here since the government doesn't care about us. The oil companies that operate near us do not care. But God has always cared for us.

Health-care services are not present in the Isohidim and Akpansung farm settlement areas. This has forced the people to consider other options, like roots and herbs, and divine healing from God. These options are situational because the people still patronize health-care service providers outside the farm settlement areas when they can afford to do so. Health-care available options in these farm settlement areas are proportional to the level of availability of health-care facilities, health-care service providers, the socioeconomic status of the people, and the natural environment of the areas.

Health-Care Intervention Programs

Health-care intervention programs are specifically strategized to solve particular health challenges. Most of these health-care intervention programs, like immunizations and other vaccinations, are targeted at children of a tender age and women. Some of the rural areas in Nigeria are randomly neglected in the quest to administer these intervention programmes. In the Isohidim and Akpansung settlement areas, participant observations gathered that there exist irregularities in the administration of special health-care intervention programs like immunizations in the areas. The majority of the study participants in their narratives confirmed the fact that health workers for immunization programmes do come into their communities once in a while for children's vaccinations. These irregularities have left these farm settlement areas to bury children who were not supposed to die in the presence of adequate health-care services.

One of the male participants from Akpansung farm settlement narrated that:

> We used to see those people with immunization vaccines coming to immunize our children once in a while. Though they do not always tell us when they will be coming so that we can keep all our children at home for the vaccinations, we tried as much as we could to call back our children from wherever they went with their mothers and those parents who did not go far from the community always brought their children for the event. But we need a health center here so that we can have access to some of these health programs.

In most rural communities where there are no health-care service providers, health intervention programs are necessary remedies for some of the health challenges facing the rural populace, especially for pregnant women and children. The majority of pregnant women according to the gathered data do not complete their antenatal processes with health-care service providers due to the distance barrier. The implication of this is that a majority of the women give birth as if we were still in the primitive era, with no trained midwives or health-care providers.

One of the female participants from the Isohidim farm settlement area in her narratives explained that:

> Pregnant women suffer a lot in this community. We have to trek to the main road before you can join vehicle to either Ukpenikang or Emmanuel Hospital at Eket. To go for antenatal visits is not easy because of the distance. When you think of what it takes to go and come back, you will find one excuse or the other to give to your husband to support your refusal to go. It is not that we wouldn't love to go, but to go and come back, it is not easy. After all, nobody wants to die or lose her baby after nine months.

Farmers and other settlers at the Isohidim and Akpansung farm settlement areas do not have access to health-care intervention programs. It was gathered that apart from immunization programs, which the vendors visit once in a long while, the areas do not have access to any other health intervention program. This depicts the fact that there is no presence of a health-care service provider in these farm settlement areas.

DISCUSSION OF FINDINGS

Most of the health-care facilities are concentrated in the urban centers of Ibeno and Esit Eket local government areas, forcing the rural dwellers to depend on other options for health care. The farm settlement areas (Isohidim and Akpansung respectively) within these local government areas are neglected in health-care facility distribution. This finding supports the position of Onokerhoraye (1999), who posited that overt attention has not been paid to equity in the planning and distribution of health-care facilities over the years in the country, and public and private health-care facilities are sporadically provided in many rural areas within the country. It was observed that there was no single health-care provider for the farmers and others in these farm settlement areas. This shows that rural farmers are neglected and abandoned in terms of health-care services and facility distribution, leading to a lack of availability of health-care services for rural farmers, especially in the farm settlement areas in AkwaIbom. The case of Isohidim and Akpansung is a pathetic one, due to the presence of multinational oil companies operating within the local government areas where they are situated. It was observed that the water used by the people for drinking and other domestic activities is coloured water due to the presence of crude oil and oil-drilling activities close to their communities.

The health challenges facing the farmers and the other dwellers found in Isohidim and Akpansung farm settlements are enormous. They range from chronic typhoid fever, malaria, measles, sore throat, hernias, and other pregnancy and infant-related diseases that lead to high mortality rates in these farm settlement areas. This finding agrees with the postulation of Hamid, Sadique, Ahmed, and Molla (2005) and Titus, Adebisola, and Adeniji (2015). According to Hamid, Sadique, Ahmed, and Molla (2005), there has been a growing recognition of the challenge of rural people's health issues and the need for it to be addressed in Nigeria. According to Titus, Adebisola, and Adeniji (2015), Nigeria still has one of the worst health indices in the world, and sadly it accounts for 10 percent of the world's maternal deaths. Most rural farmers have difficulties in access to health-care services due to the non-availability of health-care facilities in their settlement areas. It was observed that the lack of health-care facilities in farm settlement areas contributes to disease exploitation of the human race in some rural and remote areas.

Since there are no health-care facilities for easy health-care accessibility in the Isohidim and Akpansung farm settlement areas, the people resolved to use roots and herbs and trust in God for divine healing. This creates the opportunity for traditional medicine practitioners who reside at Akpansung to take wealth from the people and control the people with their claimed supernatural abilities to cure illnesses of any kind. Though people come from outside the settlement areas to patronize the traditional herbalists, the health challenges of the farmers and others in these areas still remain on the high side, as the herbalist will always find a way of explaining his inability to help with serious health issues.

Bad or poor health was discovered to have an effect on the farming activities among the famers and others in the Isohidim and Akpansung farm settlement areas. Gathered data showed that when someone is sick, he or she cannot go to farm or partake in any farming activities. This brings about a low turnover in farm produce at the end of the farming season. Findings showed that there are cases where a farmer may be ill throughout the farming season. In such a case, the farmer and his family may have to depend on the donations of other farmers for survival through the season, especially if they have spent their savings on the illness. This finding supports the position of Asenso-okyere, Chiang, Thangata, and Andam (2011) and Harper (1988). In their work, "Interactions between health and farm-labour productivity," Asenso-Okyere, Chiang, Thangata, and Andam (2011) observed that the health status of adults affects their ability to work and thus underpins the welfare of the household, including the children's development and poor health. It affects productivity at an old age and treatable problems become complicated, and sometimes lead to an untimely death when there is no access to health-care services, especially by older people. Rural Africans, like rural Black Americans, tend to perceive their health according to their ability to perform activities of daily live and not according to laboratory or X-ray findings (Harper, 1988). Most people in the Isohidim and Akpansung farm settlement areas rate their health status according to their ability to perform their farming activities on a daily basis. According to the gathered data, the good health of farmers enhances good farming activities, which brings about good agricultural turnover, and vice versa.

CONCLUSION

In the Isohidim and Akpansung farm settlement areas, located in Ibeno and EsitEket local government areas respectively, the areas are rural riverine and oil areas in Akwa Ibom State, southern Nigeria. The major source of the livelihood of the settlers is farming. According to the World Health Organization (WHO, 1948), health is a state of complete physical, mental, and social well-being and not merely the absence of disease or infirmity (Innocent, Uche, and Uche, 2014). The well-being of the farmers in these areas determines their productivity in terms of agricultural production. Availability has been a known factor that determines health-care services utilization. Where there is no availability of health-care services, as in the case of the Isohidim and Akpansung farm settlement areas, the residents resolve to depend on other options, like roots and herbs and trusting in God for divine healing. There is neither a single-room health-care centre nor a single health-care service provider found in the Isohidim and Akpansung farm settlement areas, and health-intervention programmes like immunizations have not been regular. The residents of the Isohidim and Akpansung farm settlement areas find it difficult to access health-care services. Many factors, like the absence of health-care facilities, the distance between the communities, available health-care centers, the cost of going to hospitals outside the settlements, belief in divine healing, and the availability of herbs and roots through traditional herbalists contribute to the inability of the people found in these areas to access health-care services. These have contributed to a high mortality rate in the areas, disease exploitation of the human race, and low farm productivity.

To save the people from disease exploitation, the government has to allocate health-care centers to farm settlement areas in order to boost food production toward the attainment of food security. Health-intervention programs should be made available in farm settlement areas, to alleviate the poor and bad health conditions of the farmers and their children in the areas.

REFERENCES

Aghion, P., Peter, H., Fabrice, M. (2010). "The Relationship between Health and Growth: When Lucas Meets Nelson-Phelps." *National Bureau Economic Resources* (NBER) Working Paper No. 15813.

Ajilowo, J. and Olujimi, B. (2007). Accessibility of the Rural Dwellers to Healthcare Facilities in Nigeria: The Owo Experience. *Pakistan Journal of Social Sciences*, 4(1): 44–55.

Ama, I. I., Okeme, S., & Chia, J. I. (2015). Constraints faced by Farmers in receiving Primary Healthcare Service in the North-Eastern Zone of Benue State, Nigeria. *Journal of Agricultural Economics, Environment and Social Sciences,* 1(1): 151–54. http://www.unimaid.edu.ng/jaeess.

Anderson, R. (1983). Health Services Utilization: Framework and Review. *Health Services Research*, 3: 184–99.

Anum, B. M. (2015). Acceptability and Utilization of Health Care Services among Pregnant Women in the North Central Zone of Nigeria. Unpublished master thesis.

Asenso-Okyere, K., Chiang, C., Thangata, P., and Andam, K. S. (2011). *Interactions between health and farm-labour productivity.* International Food Policy Research Institute, Washington, DC.

Bunor, P. (2004). State of Healthcare in Nigeria. Retrieved online on September 29, 2016.

Hamid, S. A., Sadique. Z., Ahmed, S., Molla, A. A. (2005). Determinants of Choice of Healthcare Providers: Evidence from Selected Rural Areas of Bangladesh. *Pakistan Journal Social Sciences,* 3(3):437–44.

Harper, M. S. (1988). Behavioural, social and mental health aspects of home care for older Americans. *Home Health Care Services Quarterly*, vol. 9, no. 4, 61–124.

Innocent, E. O., Uche, O. A., and Uche, I. (2014). Building a Solid Health Care System in Nigeria: Challenges and Prospects. http://www.mcser.org/journal/index.php/ajis/article. Retrieved on October 18, 2018.

Kajang, D. R. (2004). Organization and Management of Health Services in Nigeria: 1960–2004 (A Case Study of the Federal Ministry of Health, Abuja, Nigeria). http://stclements.edu/grad/gradkaja.pdf.

Okon, E. (2001). Change in Nigeria Health care System. The Cable. Retrieved on September 13, 2018, from https://www.thecable.ng/change-in-nigerias-healthcare-system.

Okumagba, P. O. (2011). Choice of health care services utilization by the elderly in Delta State in Nigeria. *Journal of Sociology and Anthropology*, 2(2): 131–38.

Onah, H., Ikeako, L., Iloabachie, G. (2009). Factors associated with the use of elasticity of healthcare services in Enugu, Southeastern Nigeria. *Soc. Sci. Med.*, 63(7): 1870–78.

Onokerhoraye, A. G. (1999). Access and Utilization of Modern Health Care Facilities in the Petroleum Producing Region of Nigeria: The case of Bayelsa State. Research Paper No. 162. Takemi Program in International Health Harvard School of Public Health.

Peters, D. H., Garg, A., Bloom, G., Walker, D.G., Brieger, W. R., & Rahman, M. H. (2008). Poverty and access to healthcare in developing countries. *Ann. N Y Acad. Sci.*, 1136: 161–71.

Phillips, B. S., Ononokpono, D. N., & Udofia, N. W. (2016). Complicating Causality: Patient and Professional Perspectives on Obstetric Fistula in Nigeria. *Culture, Health and Sexuality: An International Journal for Research, Intervention and Care.*

Titus, O. B., Adebisola, O. A., and Adeniji, A. O. (2015). Health-care access and utilization among rural households in Nigeria. http://www.academicjournals.org/JDAE. Retrieved on October 17, 2018.

Index

About the Editor

Aderemi Suleiman Ajala is a professor of medical anthropology, teaching in the Department of Archaeology and Anthropology, University of Ibadan, Nigeria. His research interests include culture and health, Yoruba traditional medicine, environment and health-care strategies, nationalism and politics in Nigeria, and ethnography. He is the author of *Rural Health Provisioning in Nigeria* (Peter Lang, 2009) and *Yoruba Nationalism: Culture, Politics and Violence in Southwestern Nigeria* (Rudigger Koepel, 2013). He is a recipient of several prestigious fellowships and research grants, including the British Academy Fellowship (2006); the Alexander von Humboldt Fellowship (2009); and the Rockefeller Foundation Fellowship (2011). His new research is on negotiation in culture production: the invention of human health-care strategies among the Oyo north agro-pastoral communities (2021–2023). His contact is asajala@yahoo.co.uk.

About the Contributors

Labbo Abdullahi is a senior lecturer in the Department of History, Usmanu Danfodiyo University, Sokoto, Nigeria. He has published many articles in several international and national journals and some chapters in edited books. Labbo has attended several conferences and presented many academic papers. His area of interest is the social history of medicine in northern Nigeria.

Olufunke Olufunsho Adegoke is a lecturer in the Sociology Department, University of Ibadan, Nigeria, where she received a PhD by dissertation. She researches on sociological aspects of health. Her email contact is funkeshine@gmail.com.

Olukemi K. Amodu is a professor of genetics/molecular biology and public health at the Institute of Child Health, University of Ibadan, Nigeria. She is engaged in building platforms for developing capacity in biotechnology, leveraging her core expertise in molecular genetics with a focus on bringing together clinical and biomedical scientists for public health research. Her research interests also include public health impact research, bringing health services closer to the population by providing innovative strategies for increasing vaccination demand for working mothers in the Ibadan metropolis, Nigeria.

Alex Asakitikpi was formerly a professor of sociology at Monash University, South Africa Campus, and currently is the head of the school of social science at the Independent Institute of Education (IIE MSA Campus) in Johannesburg, South Africa.

Aniekan Etim Bassey is a lecturer in the Department of Sociology and Anthropology, University of Uyo, Nigeria. He specializes in medical sociology. He can be contacted through his email at aniegem@gmail.com.

Nsere L. Danbagai is a doctoral candidate in the Department of Sociology, faculty of the social sciences, University of Ibadan, Ibadan, Nigeria. She is also a research fellow with the Institute for French Research in Africa (IFRA), based in the University of Ibadan, Nigeria. Her area of specialization is medical sociology and anthropology. Her areas of research interests are social determinants of health and the health dynamics of migrants, infectious diseases, mental health, maternal and child health, health systems, and conflict and research ethics.

Ursula V. Ette is a postgraduate student of medical sociology in the Department of Sociology and Anthropology, University of Uyo. She holds a PGDE (NOUN), PGD, Sociology and Anthropology (Uniuyo) and BNSc (Enugu). She is a registered nursing officer who specializes in anaesthesia. Presently, she is the deputy director and head of the Cinical Units of Nursing Services, University of Uyo, Teaching Hospital. Mrs. Ette is the current chairman of the National Association of Nigeria Nurses and Midwives, UUTH Chapter. Her research interests span reproductive health issues; conflicts, culture, and society; substance abuse; and other emerging topical health issues of research interest. She has contributed to many academic journals and book chapters. She is a caring mother and grandmother and is happily married to an ENT surgeon.

Ayodele S. Jegede is a professor of medical sociology/anthropology in the Department of Sociology, University of Ibadan, Nigeria. He is presently the university's research management director, having previously been the dean of the faculty of social science and the head of the Department of Sociology. He has published widely on culture and health.

Ọlálẹ́yẹ Samuel Káyọ̀dé holds a PhD degree from the University of Ibadan, Nigeria. A senior lecturer of African traditional religion with special reference to *Ifá* and the importance of *ẹbọ*-sacrifice in Yorùbá indigenous healing systems. He teaches and conducts research on *Ifá,* traditional medicine, incantation, and indigenous communication symbols.

Oyelàdé Olúfikáyọ̀ Kúnlé is a lecturer in the College of Arts, Wesley University, Ondo State, Nigeria. He obtained BA and MA degrees in religious studies, and a MSc and PhD. from the University of Ibadan. His research interests include developmental sociology, gender and development, the sociology of religion, and social ethics. He won the ISA PhD Students' Laboratory Fellowship in 2015. He is a reviewer for a number of reputable local and international journals.

Akwa Ibom State, Nigeria." He has research interests in population displacement, reproductive/maternal mortality and health, drugs and substance abuse, conflicts, culture, and society, etc. He has contributed many chapters to various books, and he has published widely in reputable local and international journals. He is happily married with three children.

Nsikanabasi Udofia Wilson is a senior lecturer in the Department of Sociology and Anthropology. She holds a PhD degree in medical anthropology from the University of Ibadan, Nigeria. She teaches anthropological aspects of health. She can be contacted at nsidofzion@yahoo.com.

Mofeyisara Oluwatoyin Omobowale is a senior research fellow at the Social and Behavioural Health Unit, Institute of Child Health, College of Medicine, University of Ibadan, Nigeria. She obtained a PhD in anthropology from the University of Ibadan, Nigeria, in 2014. She is a fellow of the American Council of Learned Societies-African Humanities Programme (2012 and 2016), Cadbury Fellowship 2014, Carnegie of New York 2016, and a short-term scholar at Brown International Advanced Research Institute (BIARI), Brown University, USA, 2013. She blends anthropological knowledge, theories, and methods in teaching and researching public health issues to impact society's well-being positively.

Paul Oluwasogo Omoniyi is a PhD candidate/research associate, Department of Sociology, University of Ibadan, with research interests in maternal and child health, women's empowerment, gender-based violence, behavioral medicine, drug/substance use prevention, mental health issues, public health, and social theory. He is a dedicated and detailed research fellow with experience in teaching, seminar presentations, and analytical and critical thinking skills.

Moses Idongesit Peters is a lecturer in the Department of Sociology and Anthropology, University of Uyo, Nigeria. He specializes in medical sociology. He can be contacted through his email: perfectakwastar@gmail.com.

Wendy Savieri is a postgraduate student at Monash University, South Africa.

Mohammed Saeed Suleiman holds a PhD in sociology and does research in medical sociology, social problems, civil society, and politics and society. He teaches at the Federal University of Gusau, Nigeria. He has contributed sufficient publications in many international and national journals and attended conferences where he has delivered papers. He can be contacted via mohammedsaeedsuleiman@gmail.com and mohammedsaeedsuleiman@fugashua.edu.ng.

Nsidibe A. Usoro is a social anthropologist and a lecturer with the Department of Sociology and Anthropology, University of Uyo, Nigeria. He holds a BSc in sociology and anthropology; an MSc. in industrial sociology, and a PhD in social anthropology (Uniuyo). He has served the university in many capacities, but currently he is the examination officer of the Sociology and Anthropology Department. Dr. Usoro carried out his anthropological fieldwork among the Bakassi returnees in Akwa Ibom state, Nigeria, between February 2015 and March 2016, where he wrote his thesis on "The Challenges of Resettlements and Re-integration of Bakassi Returnees in

Caroline Ndebia is currently a PhD student at the University of KwaZulu, Natal. She completed her master of arts degree, majoring in sociology, from Walter Sisulu University in South Africa. Her area of interest is health and well-being in society.

Emeka E. Obioha is a full professor of sociology and a faculty chair of research and higher degrees in the FHSSL at Walter Sisulu University, South Africa. He has extensive expertise in academic and community-engaged applied research in institutional development capabilities, social control, and social systems equilibrium analysis. Emeka is a United Nations (UN) expert in social and development affairs, a member of United Nations office of the special adviser on Africa (UN-OSAA)—Knowledge Network.

Chigozirim Ogubuike is a doctoral student at the Institute of Child Health, University of Ibadan, Nigeria. She is a results-oriented public health professional with experience in both quantitative and qualitative research. She is passionate about innovation and strategic solutions, and she is culturally and socially sensitive, is technologically savvy, and can adapt to multiple and changing demands. Her research interest is in child and adolescent health, sexual and reproductive health, family research, contemporary issues, public health research, gender variations, and women's health. She is a young researcher and open to fellowship opportunities, research funding, and further training.

Janet Ogundairo is a PhD student at the Department of Sociology, University of Ibadan, Nigeria, and a research fellow with the French Institute for Research in Africa (IFRA), Nigeria. Her research interests include the anthropology of pastoralism; conflicts; health-care delivery systems; and migration. Janet is also interested in the sociological and anthropological perspective of antimicrobial resistance. She has scholarly outputs in journal articles and book chapters published by reputable publishing outfits.

Ayotunde Olayori Oguntade holds the following degrees: DTh, BTh (NBTS, Ogbomoso), BA in Christian religious studies (Ajayi Crowther University, Oyo), MTh (NBTS), MA (University of Jos) and PhD (NBTS). He lectures in the Department of Intercultural Studies, faculty of theological studies, Nigerian Baptist Theological Seminary, Ogbomoso (NBTS), and he is also the director of archives and museums. He is a member of the Nigerian Association of Church History and Musicological Studies (NACHAMS) and Sacred Earth Ministry. He has published articles in both national and international journals and has contributed some chapters in books in his areas of interest: church history, missions, and world religions.

www.ingramcontent.com/pod-product-compliance
Lightning Source LLC
Chambersburg PA
CBHW051256200926
51612CB00002B/62
* 9 7 8 1 6 6 6 9 3 9 8 6 6 *